Negotiating Ageing

The world is growing older and this is a historically unprecedented phenomenon. Negotiating such change, personally, socially and for governments and international organisations requires an act of cultural adaptation. Two key questions arise: What is the purpose of a long life? and How do we adapt to societies where generations are of approximately the same size? A number of pre-existing narratives can be identified; however, it is argued that contemporary policies have produced a premature answer which may eclipse the potential arising from lifecourse change.

In this book Simon Biggs discusses ways of interrogating these questions and the adaptations we make to them. Four major areas, all of which have been suggested as solutions to population ageing, are critically assessed, including work, spirit, body and family. Areas covered include the mixed evidence on work as an answer, the relationship between work, ageing and health, narratives of spirit, belief and wisdom, the body and the natural, anti-ageing medicine, critical approaches to dementia, plus family and intergenerational relations.

This book is particularly useful for those trying to make sense of population ageing and negotiate solutions. It describes a number of concepts that can be used to assess what we are told about a long life and how generations can adapt together.

With the cultural landscape moving away from traditional interpretations of old age, the question of adult ageing is of growing interest to a number of groups. This book is essential reading for social and health-care workers, other helping professionals, policy makers, social scientists and all who encounter the prospect of a long life.

Simon Biggs' interests include the relationship between social identity and adult ageing, including an analysis of international and national social policy and the dynamics of a changing adult lifecourse. He is Professor of Gerontology and Social Policy in the School of Social & Political Sciences at the University of Melbourne and runs a research group on inclusive ageing at the Australian social justice charity, The Brotherhood of St Laurence. He has worked as a Community Psychologist and for the UK Social Work Council. From 2004 to 2010 he was Director of the Institute of Gerontology, King's College London UK. He has been a founding member of the World Economic Forum's Global Agenda Council on Ageing Societies (2008 to 2014) and has liaised with EU, UK, Australian and Canadian Governments on population ageing, dignity in later life and elder protection. He is currently an Adviser to the Danish Center for Applied Social Science. In 2016 he was elected a Fellow of the British Academy of Social Science. Simon has a number of continuing international links including the Universities of Helsinki and Kings College London. His PhD is in Psychology, from Birkbeck College, London. He has published widely including the book, *Generational Intelligence* with Ariela Lowenstein (Routledge 2011).

Routledge Key Themes in Health and Society

www.routledge.com/Routledge-Key-Themes-in-Health-and-Society/book-series/
RKTHS

Available titles include

The Story of Nursing in British Mental Hospitals
Echoes from the corridors
Niall McCrae and Peter Nolan

Living with Mental Disorder
Insights from qualitative research
Jacqueline Corcoran

A New Ethic of 'Older'
Subjectivity, surgery and self-stylization
Bridget Garnham

Social Theory and Nursing
Edited by Martin Lipscomb

Older Citizens and End-of-Life Care
Social work practice strategies for adults in later life
Malcolm Payne

Digital Technologies and Generational Identity
ICT usage across the life course
Sakari Taipale, Terhi-Anna Wilksa and Chris Gilleard

Partiality and Justice in Nursing Care
Marita Nordhaug

Negotiating Ageing
Cultural adaptation to the prospect of a long life
Simon Biggs

Negotiating Ageing

Cultural Adaptation to the Prospect
of a Long Life

Simon Biggs

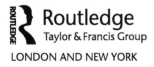

LONDON AND NEW YORK

First published 2018 by Routledge

2 Park Square, Milton Park, Abingdon, Oxfordshire OX14 4RN
52 Vanderbilt Avenue, New York, NY 10017

Routledge is an imprint of the Taylor & Francis Group, an informa business

First issued in paperback 2019

British Library Cataloguing-in-Publication Data
A catalogue record for this book is available from the British Library

Library of Congress Cataloging-in-Publication Data
A catalog record for this book has been requested

ISBN: 978-1-138-94775-7 (hbk)
ISBN: 978-0-367-43101-3 (pbk)

Typeset in Times New Roman
by Apex CoVantage, LLC

To Irja, Guy and Eve

Contents

Foreword   viii
Acknowledgements   xi

1 The prospect of a long life   1

2 Interrogating personal and intergenerational ageing   14

3 Work to the rescue?   28

4 Is work good or bad for health?   46

5 Spirit, belief and the in-between   62

6 Lifecourse, gerotranscendence and wisdom   80

7 The ageing body, the social and the natural   97

8 Anti-ageing   112

9 Dementia   128

10 Family and generations   148

Conclusions   167

Index   176

Foreword

We negotiate ageing in many ways, and we are simultaneously encouraged to run our lives according to a number of narratives, scripts or, as Dan McAdams has said, 'stories to live by'. This is no less true for midlife and beyond as it is for other narrative scripts to do with gender, childhood or culture. And as the lifecourse grows longer and there are more people of mature age about, the ways open to us to negotiate a passage through the lifecourse and with other generational groups become increasingly important. These twin challenges – negotiating the prospect of a long life in circumstances where generations are becoming approximately the same size – take us from considering demographic changes to questions of cultural adaptation. How should we live in societies that include many more older adults and are increasingly intergenerationally complex?

This book is principally concerned with ageing, and it is narratives of adult ageing that take priority over others. Here, the need for cultural adaptation is par-ticularly acute, as the personal and social scripts we have to hand are more often than not drawn from other parts of the lifecourse or other priority areas than that of lifecourse change. Also, it seems like the reliability of many other areas is either in flux or under considerable strain. These would include the fields of economics, climate change, health, trust in the global financial system, and concern over rising social inequality. As a student once said to me, 'I thought ageing was boring, but now I see it affects everything!'

While this book cannot do justice to all of these global concerns, it is worth noting that, like climate change, population ageing is a 'slow burn' issue; the effects take time to become visible and are often met with the twin responses of panic or indifference. In many ways, it is an unthought-known of the day-to-day. Chris Bollas has used this term to refer to things that we all 'know', often at a preconscious level, but do not think about in everyday life. When it comes to ageing, the reasons that the knowns of adult ageing are generally pushed aside may include a fear of personal ageing, resistance towards one's own parents, devaluation of citizens who are considered unproductive, envy of an escape from the pressures of earlier life stages, fear of poverty and an inability to deal culturally and personally with the vulnerability of the human condition. As Car-roll Estes reminds us here, the personal is intimately connected to the social and the structural.

Negotiation itself requires creating a critical distance between ourselves and the stories we are being encouraged to live by. Stepping back from the storyline allows us to evaluate it rather than being absorbed by it as the only possible way of living with longevity and intergenerational connection. Negotiation is therefore premised on the possibility of finding options rather than immersion in pre-existing assumptions. The narratives that are described and critically assessed in this book include work, spirit, the body and family. Each has at some time been presented as an answer to the purpose for a long life, and while some such discourses appear to close down our options, others seem to open them up.

The book begins with two introductory chapters. One outlines current demographic and cultural trends and examines how the 'problem of ageing' has been perceived. A second covers the particular orientation that informs the arguments that follow. It suggests some conceptual tools that might help in making sense of contemporary ageing. Two chapters then critically assess whether work can come to the rescue as a solution to the public problems associated with extra years of life. Here, Chapter 4 critically examines the policy push towards longer working lives and evidence on what younger and older workers want. Chapter 5 then looks at the relationship between health, continued work and retirement. Here the answer seems to be that while extra years of healthy life can allow longer years of work, work in itself is not necessarily healthy. After work, Chapters 6 and 7 address approaches to the spirit. This section poses a very different set of questions: the initial chapter asks what different belief systems and spirituality say about a long life, old age and intergenerational relations. The following chapter examines questions of transformation, liminality and the concepts of wisdom and gerotranscendence. Discourses of the spirit appear to address questions of 'in between-ness' and vulnerability that inclusion through working life cannot. Chapters 8, 9 and 10 address the body as a site of physical and mental change, raising questions of naturalness and how biological elements of ageing have been conceived. Two issues are then examined in greater detail: the hope associated with anti-ageing medicine and the fears associated with dementia. Both are placed in a social context in which particular narrative structures shape our understanding of the potential of a long life and of personal futures. These chapters examine the interconnective relationship between understandings of the biological and the social in considering a long life and intergenerational relationships. A final chapter concerns generation, most commonly expressed through the family. Families sit at the crossroads of the public and private spheres and cannot be understood, it is argued, without looking at their connection to wider social and historical phenomena. The way that family is used to both contain emotional aspects of ageing and balance twin tensions between informal care and state support are critically assessed.

In the last section, tentative conclusions are drawn on the value of a long life and their implications for intergenerational relations. In addition to new themes, this section reconnects with and interprets work undertaken by the author, Ariela Lowenstein and Irja Haapala on generational intelligence.

This book is not primarily descriptive; rather, it is used to pursue an argument about contemporary thinking on adult ageing and intergenerational relationships.

This argument lies behind the analysis and evidence supplied. It goes something like this: contemporary preoccupations with labour economics, work and the economy are an insufficient basis on which to judge the value and purpose of a long life. An alternative material basis lies, in front of us but unseen, in the inherent phases and rhythms of the human lifecourse. These require personal and social negotiation, and each phase has its own contribution to make. In a period where many of the cultural markers for longevity and population ageing are in flux, it is important to re-examine the interaction between social, psychological and biological aspects of ageing both to evaluate existing narratives and to invent new ones. While it is difficult to predict the possibilities inherent in a long life until one actually gets there, as individuals and as populations, it may be possible to examine the advantages and disadvantages of the narratives already in play and thereby sketch out the spaces in which new understandings can take shape.

Acknowledgements

I would like to thank Irja Haapala-Biggs for her unfailing support, her debate on the argument pursued in this book and, not least, her work on dementia and the final manuscript. I would also like to acknowledge Thubauld Moulaert, Michael McGann and Ashley Carr for continued discussion and debate on issues to do with work in later life and anti-ageing approaches; older workers, retirement and work-life balance; and residential and dementia care respectively. Also due thanks are Elizabeth Ozanne, Antti Karisto and Ariela Lowenstein for their contributions to the development of my gerontological thinking and continued belief in the direction that has been taken.

Finally, I would like to thank the directors and staff of the Leyden Academy on Vitality & Ageing for their kindness and support while part of this book was written.

1 The prospect of a long life

Key themes

- Shifting perspectives from demographic change to cultural adaptation
- Balancing reflection and engagement as priorities for a long life
- The role of policy in shifts from holistic to particular forms of legitimacy
- Managing cultural and personal uncertainty
- Increasing precarity across the lifecourse as a source of generational solidarity
- The need for a critical approach

This first chapter identifies some of the key elements that are shaping contemporary thinking about adult ageing. It takes as its starting point the rapid demographic changes that have marked the transition from the twentieth to the twenty-first centuries and goes on to explore how changes in the relative numbers of older and younger adults have been accompanied by cultural shifts in the meaning of a long life. These changes are a global phenomenon, embracing developing and developed, emerging and mature, and poorer and richer economies and societies. This gives rise to two fundamental questions. The first asks what the purpose of a long life might be. The second asks how societies will adapt from a world in which there were relatively few elders and many younger people to one in which generations are approximately the same size. It is suggested that contemporary social and public policies have produced a premature answer that may eclipse the potential arising from lifecourse change. This has implications for a critical approach to ageing societies and a rethinking of critiques and solutions based primarily on economic participation rather than lifecourse priorities. These issues and their possible alternatives will be examined in detail as the book progresses.

Global ageing

In 2050, the global population aged over 60 will reach two billion, making this age group three times larger than it was in 2000 (United Nations, 2016). This is a challenge that is facing both mature and emerging economies, and the debate on the future shape of a long life is one that is key to social development in the 21st century. It is increasingly exercising the minds of policy makers, service providers and generational groups throughout the world. And whilst living longer and, for many, healthier older lives is a cause for celebration, it has, as the 21st century emerges from the shadow of the twentieth, increasingly been reframed as a social, economic and political problem. In 2012, the World Economic Forum (Beard et al., 2012) Global Risks group identified population ageing as one of the top five issues facing the world community in terms of international stability. The others were climate change, migration, social inequality and pandemics. Harvard-based economic demographers Bloom, Canning and Lubet (2015) have argued that as the challenges of population ageing 'come from the fact that our current institutional and social arrangements are unsuited for ageing populations and shifting demographics; our proposed solution is therefore to change our institutions and social arrangements' (2015: 86).

If, as the WEF implies, the task of addressing global ageing is principally one of cultural adaptation, the question arises: Which adaptations suit which interests? The forms that adaptation takes therefore require critical consideration.

The changing promise of a long life

The speed with which our attitudes to adult ageing have changed can be seen by a series of events held by the United Nations (UN). The UN has held two World Assemblies on ageing, one in Vienna in 1982 and a second in Madrid in 2002. Both assemblies attempted to define the essential role of older adults in society, and it is interesting to look at the differences between the two. The first stated that

> A longer life provides humans with an opportunity to examine their lives **in retrospect**, to correct some of their mistakes, to get closer to the truth and **to achieve a different understanding** of the sense and value of their actions.
> (Vienna International Plan of Action on Ageing, 1982)

While Article 10 of the second says,

> The potential of older persons is a powerful basis for **future development**. This enables society to rely increasingly on the skills, experience and wisdom of older persons, not only to take the lead in their own betterment but also to **participate actively** in that of **society** as a whole.
> (Madrid International Plan of Action on Ageing, 2002)

Twenty years is a relatively short time in historical terms, yet the tenor of the descriptions show a markedly different approach to the relationship between personal ageing and society. A couple of the key words in each have been put into bold type to illustrate the change in expectations of later life. The form of social inclusion envisaged by the two statements varies significantly. One appears as a personal, reflective task, looking across the lifecourse via a sifting of accrued experience; the second privileges the application of particular skills in the here and now, as a springboard for future aspiration.

While we are still waiting, at the time of writing, for a third international plan, there have been a number of other statements, perhaps most clearly articulated by the European Union. In 2012, The European Year of Active Ageing and Intergenerational Solidarity made the following announcement:

> Empowering older people to age in good health and to contribute more actively to the labour market and to their communities will help us cope with our demographic challenge in a way that is fair and sustainable for all generations.
>
> (European Union, 2012)

There are many things worth noting about the European Year, but what stands out is a narrowing of the aspirational tone of 2002, to a much more sharply focussed role for older adults. The contribution of older adults is to be channelled into work and work-like activities, such as volunteering.

The degree to which these differing statements reflect changing historical and economic conditions is retrospectively much easier to see than it was at the time. And perhaps the first 'Vienna' version itself reflects what Piketty (2014) has called the 'trentes glorieuses' or thirty years of growth and development of health and welfare services that followed the end of the World War II. Certainly in the West, this was seen as a period of growing prosperity and late life as a well-earned release from the rigours of working life. The second 'Madrid' statement is very much the child of those years of social improvement but focussing on the contribution that a fitter and wealthier older population might make. Its holism reflected the views of the World Health Organization (WHO), characterising 'active ageing' (WHO, 2002) as an opportunity to develop a whole raft of potential that older adults had still to develop. Indeed, the thirty years between 1950 and 1979 could be seen as a time of clearing away the risks to allow a flourishing of the majority of western populations.

The recessional world of the second decade of the twenty-first century is reflected in the 2012 statement. Here, the developmental potential of a long life has been reigned in. It has been corralled in the service of extrinsic priorities, mostly to do with labour economics. A long life is not to be viewed as a period of multiple purposes and diverse social contributions but as a pool of potential workers, which will hopefully restore profitability to an ailing world economy.

While these statements point to alternative visions of a long life with implications for the contributions made by different generational groups, it is also possible to see the UN declarations as two sides of a coin. They may not be paths towards either disengagement or to active ageing but simultaneous developments of reflection and engagement, which perhaps illustrate interior and exterior orientations to the task of growing older. They reflect how one responds to personal lifecourse change and how one can connect to the social world.

Both visions appear threatened by public rhetoric that stokes generational competition, with material productivity as the principal criterion by which to gain social legitimacy. At the time of writing, both of these trends have marked a recessional and neo-recessional world characterised by extreme economic inequality and a tendency to use generational rivalry as a distraction from these deeper concerns.

The UN are now only one of a growing number of international organisations that circulate briefings, bulletins and working papers on ageing populations, which also include the WHO, the Organisation for Economic Cooperation & Development (OECD), the International Labour Organisation (ILO), the World Bank and even the Central Intelligence Agency (CIA). Each explores a different consequence of population ageing and promotes a particular ideological position.

In social terms, there are certainly indications that a long life in the twenty-first century is becoming increasingly precarious. The ILO's World Social Protection Report 2014/15, for example, indicates that 49% of all people over pensionable age do not receive a pension and for many who do, pension levels may leave them below national poverty lines. Additionally, future pensioners will receive lower pensions in at least 14 European countries, whilst in the United States, a reliance on private schemes, housing wealth and stocks and shares have increased the risk of poverty in old age.

What emerges from these changing perspectives is that expectations of a long life have become increasingly contested, and the notion of the purpose and contribution of older adults is itself in a state of cultural flux.

Demographic certainties

So what are these demographic changes that have provoked so many twists and turns in the ways we are expected to view growing old and living longer lives?

The analysis of population ageing has been characterised by three defining demographic facts. People are living longer. Generations or age groups are becoming approximately the same size. And the oldest old are the group growing most quickly. It is now a commonplace political and economic debate that we are moving from a demographic triangle to a column. That is to say that in traditional societies, where a lot of children are born but die relatively quickly and with many adults also dying in early midlife, through poor health care, during childbirth and the greater likelihood of physical threats and accidents, the population profile tapers off pretty quickly, with only a few elders surviving to the top of the age pyramid. Under current conditions, however, people are having fewer children and living longer, which will eventually create a population in which each age group is of approximately the same size. This latter pattern, because of its historical uniqueness, leaves us with few tools to understand its implications and ways in which to respond.

These 'facts of ageing' rest on a series of underlying demographic changes (United Nations, 2016). The first concerns declining global fertility, measured by the number of children born per woman. This has fallen from 5 children in 1950 to approximately 2.5 today and is projected to fall to 2 by 2050. The most rapid descent is expected to occur in developing countries, halving between 1965 and 2050. Second is increased longevity, the average number of years lived, which is set to increase globally from 48 to 75, from 1950 to 2050. While there are disparities between mature and emerging economies – with wealthy industrial countries rising on average to 82 years, this is no longer a local phenomenon. In fact, when the speed at which developing countries' or emerging economies' demographics are changing is taken into account, it is apparent these nations are ageing much more rapidly than others. If the UN definition of an ageing society is accepted, when 14% of the population reach 60 years and over, then the longest time is estimated to have occurred in France, at over a hundred years, whereas Thailand and the Philippines are expected to make the same transition in as little as twenty years. Over time, a fall in mortality and a fall in births plus an increase in longevity radically reshapes the age structure of a society and leads to the column shape we are now achieving.

These changes affect the proportion of working to non-working people in a population, commonly referred to as the dependency ratio, spawning a series of apocalyptic predictions of doom – for productivity, health-care systems and social wages, such as pensions. However, as Beard et al. (2012) point out, such calls of woe have happened before and are 'strongly reminiscent of the work by Paul Ehrlich and the Club of Rome in the late 1960s, which predicted mass starvation and human misery in the 1970s and 1980s as a result of rapid population growth, or what was termed "the population bomb"' (2012: 4).

The world population did double from three to six million from 1960 to 2000. However, technological advances and levels of education increased dramatically, and per capita income increased by 115%. The world as we knew it had not ended, although it had changed radically.

Bloom et al. (2015) point out that, in terms of dependency ratios, increasing numbers of people leaving the workforce as they achieve late life are largely offset by a reduced youth dependency ratio marked by fewer younger dependents, even though they are spending a longer amount of time in education rather than in work. In the United States, the ratio had grown from seventeen adults aged 65 and over (per one hundred working-aged adults) in 1980 to twenty-one by 2013. However, the same ratio for younger people under 15 had fallen from thirty-four to twenty-nine. Neither is it clear that older adults are a net cost on younger generations. At least in the private sphere, generational transfers tend to travel from older to younger family members, even in later life (Irwin, 1998). In a 2011 communique, the OECD has noted that in the public sphere there may actually be a form of fiscal generational altruism associated with large infrastructural investments, where the contributors may not live long enough to receive the full benefit of investments made. It has also been argued that it may be incorrect to assume that continued working is the solution to the fiscal costs of health, for example, if 60% of tax revenue is raised outside taxable income (Betts, 2014). So while the figures for demographic change are by now well known, their implications have yet to be fully worked through and may not conform to widespread negative expectations.

Cultural uncertainties

It has become common to suggest that an ageing population is a policy priority. What is less commonly recognised is that this is not simply a question of demographic change and economic response, it is also one of cultural meaning and the possibilities attributed to adult ageing and later life.

Mature aged individuals have in the immediate past become generally richer and fitter than preceding generations (Metz & Underwood, 2005). As a result, many have developed lifestyles that reflect a mixture of extended youthful activities and novel mature priorities. This conclusion has been supported by longstanding evidence of a compression of morbidity, meaning that people are living longer and also healthier lives until their final years (Fries, 1980), that decrements associated with old age are increasingly modifiable and sometimes reversible (Rowe & Kahn, 1987), and by the growth of occupational pensions (Phillipson, 1998). While each of these points have since been contested, they are still the bedrock for thinking in this area. In the late 20th and early 21st centuries, we have moved, it is argued, from an understanding based on late-life dependency to one that sees older people as potentially active consumers or continuing producers or some combination of both. So, while there are particular concerns about the numbers and distribution of older adults in various national populations, there is also a common understanding that generally speaking there are not only more older people about but they are healthier and more financially independent than had been the case in previous historical periods. This, it has been argued, produced a blurring of life stages and functional ageing, so that different generations are becoming increasingly the same (Featherstone & Hepworth, 1989), and a set of lifestyles have emerged that have separated patterns of consumption from traditional conceptions of age as decline (Gilleard & Higgs, 2005). If one were to try to encapsulate this as a cultural trend, it may be possible to say that 'Everyone wants to live a long life, but no one wants to grow old'.

For societies to successfully respond, to make this transition work, a number of modifications have been suggested, including a re-design of our cities (WHO, 2007), the extension of healthy life years (Olshansky, 2007), intergenerational negotiation of roles and expectations (Biggs & Lowenstein, 2011) and a re-evaluation of the contribution of older adults to the societies in which they live (Walker, 2009).

Personal ageing and the effects of population change have also become associated with a series of nagging uncertainties. How is one to come to terms with both the probability of longer life and the certainty of running out of personal existence? What are the legitimate social roles made available to longevity and intergenerational relationships? Which policies and professional practices can best respond to shifts in population requirements? As one grows older, the prospect of a long life exists in a paradoxical relationship between a trajectory of increasing certainty, in that life's ending is now on the horizon, and uncertainty, in that one does not know when, what sort of life quality one can expect and how wider social expectations will tip the balance in one direction or another. Cultural responses to ageing become increasingly important when placed in the light of Baltes and Baltes' (1990) observation that at the beginnings and endings of life, the balance changes from reliance on personal, biological and physical autonomy to interde-pendence between social actors and cultural supports. In other words, while most people can rely on their bodies to see them through to a feeling of independence in the middle years, in childhood and old age, they rely on the kindness of others.

Tension between the certainties and uncertainties of ageing has a number of implications for the way we see growing older and the value of intergenerational relationships. An advantage, at least in terms of being able to put oneself in the shoes of the age-other, is the natural inevitability that if we are lucky enough, we will all grow old. A transmutation into the age-other over time occurs, so that each of us has a personal interest in the social conditions of ageing. However, a disad-vantage lies in a fear of the consequences of the process of ageing. Ageing can be seen as a 'bad thing' from the perspective of youth and midlife, giving rise to the dynamics of rejecting potentialities nascent within the future self and projecting disadvantages onto other people who come to signify those unwanted futures. You can then reject unwelcome prospects from a distance. If old age becomes associ-ated with poverty and unmet dependence or a sense of consumerist excess, then to denigrate older adults, to both express one's frustration and symbolically evacu-ate any personal threat, becomes a psychological possibility. There is, of course, a positive side to adult ageing – greater maturity, ability to more readily perceive systems and bigger pictures, more developed social skills, and being less prey to emotional and hormonal imperatives. However, the dominant social attitude, in industrial and postindustrial societies, is negative.

An additional source of uncertainty arises from a simultaneous experiencing of the erosion of current and future life chances. Both youth and age are becoming more precarious. Guy Standing (2011) has argued that the processes of increasing globalisation have created a precarity in everyday life, marked by job insecurity, discontinuity of identity and lack of time control. These, he suggests, would par-ticularly affect young adults who may well have an education but find themselves in work that has little security, poor pay and no obvious career pathway. There are certainly indications that a long life is also becoming a precarious one, including The International Labour Organisation's World Social Protection Report 2014/15 (2015), cited above, and the Australian BSL Social Exclusion Monitor (2014). According to the monitor, in a country that has one of the highest standards of living in the world, 15% of 55- to 64-year-olds were living below the income-poverty line (defined as 50% of the median equivalent household disposable income), and the level of disadvantage goes up with age. The likelihood of an increasingly precarious ageing would be exacerbated by policies aimed at lengthened statutory retirement ages and questions over availability and forms of work, plus inadequate or unaffordable care and support services (Biggs, 2014). A key consequence of this changing landscape would be that there may no longer be the predictabil-ity to a long life that many in advanced economies had come to expect. Taken together these trends leave us in an uncertain world where the prospect of a long life becomes increasingly difficult to navigate. They not only raise the possibility of a return to old age marked by social disadvantage and poverty; they also suggest that generations not yet in old age will have little chance to build the securities that previously arose from decent work and a supportive state. As such a fight against precarity forms a common site for generational solidarity, now and for intergenerationally workable futures. Further, it is a social phenomenon; it is the product of policies that can be changed. It is not rooted in the biology of an ageing of the body but has consequences that both exacerbate the likelihood and ability to handle disability in later life.

The cumulative effect of these trends acts as a provocation. We must learn to critically understand the ways in which adaptation to population ageing is being described and put it in the context of a personal experience of ageing and its implications for intergenerational relations.

A critical approach

Questions surrounding adult ageing set us down at the crossroads of our structural and personal worlds. They provoke us to interrogate the uncertainties and certainties of a long life.

Gerontological ideas can act as a tool to understand the world and ultimately act upon it. And the way we do that depends greatly on the historical and personal circumstances we find ourselves thrown into. In many ways, they are a route out of being determined by events. They allow us to stand back and try to work out what is going on. And in this way, they help us determine what to do about it, with whom and in which direction. It affects our interior as well as exterior worlds – the ways we think about our own ageing, our interaction with others and the factors that determine our life circumstances. When seen in this way, to say that a concern with ideas is some sort of exercise in idle navel gazing, preferably from a tower built of unsustainable and endangered animal parts, is a significant misunderstanding. In fact, one might even go so far as to say it is a wilful misunderstanding of the relationship between conceptualisation, practical action and social change. When Bob Butler said that gerontology was an amalgam of science and advocacy (in Moody, 2001) he was in part alluding to how closely gerontology followed current events and used its evidence base to promote the interests of older adults. Reading his comments through Foucault (1976/1981), we know that power and knowledge are never entirely separable, as politics influences which research is considered relevant, and it is often also a question of which voice is dominant, who is advocating for whom and in which direction. For social gerontology, the relationship between social policy and the expectations placed on us as we grow old has always been a vexed one, and as Caroll Estes (2001) in the United States and Chris Phillipson (2012) in the UK have repeatedly reminded us, it is contingent on structural inequalities that interact intimately with people's everyday lives.

A conceptual journey

My own theoretical position has evolved over time, starting from a combination of psychosocial, political-economic and social-constructionist approaches in order to understand the relationship between what is tacit and what is explicit in social relationships and the conditions experienced by older adults. This crystallised around how personal experience interacted with developments in social policy and other less formal social narratives, such as those popularly associated with adult ageing and the lifecourse. I suppose it has always been marked by a concern with the degree of autonomy social actors can exert and how forms of positive relationship and collective engagement can be achieved. This interest often became associated with barriers to self- and collective expression, such as social ageism and, in its most extreme form, elder abuse. It became clearer to me that the strategies people used to manage their everyday identities were closely connected to their experience of ageing in others and in themselves. Rather than being caught in a war with their own bodies (Featherstone & Hepworth, 1989), I saw the core contradiction being between a mature imagination that could not be expressed and social attitudes that shaped the legitimising forms of expression that were made available to them (Biggs, 1999). As mainstream social policy began to catch up with many of the proposals made by critical gerontology, at least in terms of content – age being not simply a matter of biological decline, no compulsory retirement age, and the recognition of age discrimination and elder abuse as explicit social problems, for example – it became clear that a new form of critique, paying greater attention to process rather than content, was needed. A process of age-imperialism (Biggs, 2004) appeared to take place whereby the life-priorities of one group were colonised by priorities from elsewhere, from other, more dominant age groups or from extrinsic social and economic forces. The co-option and accompanying distortion of once radical concepts to justify the privatisation of social welfare and erosion of pension security, the requirement to work rather than the option of staying working, and the increasing uncertainty that a new policy turn was bringing to ageing in mature economies made it a priority to re-evaluate what a contemporary critical approach to ageing might be. This made me increasingly aware of the interdependence between power-knowledge and legitimising narratives, shaped by times that restricted social value to ones that were economic and instrumental, which, in turn, led to a re-examination of the processes that allowed older people to be both marginal and a growing subject for public debate. At the interpersonal level, this showed itself as a lack of empathic understanding of the age-other and a need for greater generational intelligence. Ariela Lowenstein and I (2011) both saw intergenerational relations as a great source of strength and of misunderstanding, which could easily become, as Martin Kohli (2005) had suggested, a new field on which wider political and economic rivalries would be played out – not that they are themselves a source of inequality, but as a cloak, covering deeper contradictions within society.

My thinking here, as with a number of other critical gerontologists (Dillaway & Byrnes, 2009; Calasanti & King, 2011; Martinson & Halpern, 2011; see Van Dyk, 2014 for a review), paid renewed attention to the discontinuities, or changes, that characterise a life lived over a long time. Continuities that had driven earlier critical thinking – staying in work, avoiding bodily ageing, social inclusion – appeared less and less satisfying, both intellectually and as a solution to the question of cultural adaptation. The roots of positive change lie in new priorities suggested by different stages of life and existential questions that become increasingly pressing as one can no longer avoid the fact that life is finite, as well as in the cumulative deprivations and advantages that affected different social groups. A key element of this approach draws on psychosocial understandings of changing priorities that face adults as they grow older (Jung, 1932/1967; Tornstam, 2007; Dittman-Kohli & Joop, 2007). While people generally sought continuity of identity, then, they also required discontinuity of priority to engage in more personally relevant forms of ageing and change. The way one engages with these processes of change should affect the degree to which the self is in harmony with inherent lifecourse priorities and is able to express parts of the self that might otherwise be suppressed. A more adaptive identity lies in an agentic tension, created between personal and social experience and the possibilities for what remains hidden and what can be expressed. In social situations, this tension expresses itself in a need to connect with others and also protect oneself from damaging attack.

It was striking how quickly traditionally critical policy issues had been absorbed by mainstream policy making, but in ways that were hardly of most people's choosing. The material base, as manifested by economics, had proven an insecure and shifting surface on which alone to build a lasting critique of contemporary ageing in society. The materiality of economics itself needed anchoring in something equally concrete, which from a psychosocial perspective, arose from that experience of lifecourse change itself.

Two questions

This trajectory led me to thinking that at root two questions arise when demographic shifts are considered alongside personal and cultural adaptation. These two questions are as follows:

- What is the purpose of a long life?
- How do we adapt to a society where generations will be approximately the same size?

It is clear from the above that as a global society we have to adapt and that this is not so much a demographic as a cultural task. For social gerontology, in particular, the question that arises is what sort of adaptation should we be aiming for? What, in other words, might the relationship between lifecourse continuity and discontinuity, personal experience and social structures, be? And how is it reflected in wider social discourse on the purpose of a long life?

From a policy and professional point of view, these questions often boil down to 'What to do with all those older folk?' and 'How will the generations get along?' It is suggested in this book that the first appears to have achieved an international consensus that is currently of hegemonic proportions. Both nationally and internationally, the accepted answer is to make people work longer (Moulaert & Biggs, 2013). The second appears at the time of writing to be in transition, reflecting a historical stage in the evolution of more complex gerontological understanding about ageing and social change.

The problem with the international consensus is that it may be premature. It may simply be an import from other life phases, driven by extrinsic priorities and a quick fix, which really does not constitute cultural adaptation at all. Rather it imposes a 'more of the same' response whereby pre-existing priorities trump creative alternatives. It is, in this sense, an act of premature closure that eclipses or denies lifecourse change and the specific meaning of a long life.

In an attempt to answer those questions – how best to adapt culturally and socially to a world where generations are approximately the same size, and what might be the purpose of a long life – a number of answers will be looked at. These include ideas around work, spirituality, the body, and family, each of which has been suggested as a way to interpret adult ageing. Some of the tools that can be used to interrogate these debates are elaborated in the next chapter.

References

Baltes, P. B., & Baltes, M. M. (1990). Psychological perspectives on successful aging: The model of selective optimization with compensation. In P. B. Baltes & M. M. Baltes (Eds.), *Successful aging: Perspectives from the behavioral sciences* (pp. 1–34). New York, NY: Cambridge University Press.

Beard, J., Biggs, S., Bloom, D., Fried, L., Hogan, P., Kalache, A., & Olshansky, J. (2012). *Global population ageing: Peril or promise?* (Working Paper No. 89). Geneva, Switzerland: World Economic Forum.

Betts, K. (2014). The ageing of the Australian population: Triumph or disaster? Retrieved May 8, 2017, from www.swinburne.edu.au/news/latest-news/2014/05/reaping-the-benefits-of-an-ageing-population.php

Biggs, S. (1999). *The mature imagination: Dynamics of identity in midlife and beyond.* Buckingham, England: Open University Press.

Biggs, S. (2004). New ageism: Age imperialism, personal experience and ageing policy. In S.-O. Daatland & S. Biggs (Eds.), *Ageing and diversity: Multiple pathways and cultural migrations* (pp. 95–106). Bristol, England: Policy Press.

Biggs, S. (2014). Adapting to an ageing society, the need for cultural change. *Policy Quarterly, 10*(3), 12–17.

Biggs, S., & Lowenstein, A. (2011). *Generational intelligence: A critical approach to age relations.* New York, NY: Routledge.

Bloom, D. E., Canning, D., & Lubet, A. (2015). Global population aging: Facts, challenges, solutions & perspectives. *Daedalus, 144*(2), 80–92.

Brotherhood of St Laurence Social Exclusion Monitor. Retrieved August 1, 2014, from www.bsl.org.au/knowledge/social-exclusion-monitor/

Calasanti, T., & King, N. (2011). A feminist lens on the third age: Refining the framework. In D. C. Carr & K. Komp (Eds.), *Gerontology in the era of the third age* (pp. 67–85). New York, NY: Springer Publishing Company.

Dillaway, H., & Byrnes, M. (2009). Reconsidering successful aging: A call for renewed and expanded academic critiques and conceptualizations. *Journal of Applied Gerontology, 28*(6), 702–722.

Dittman-Kohli, F., & Joop, D. (2007). Self and life management. In J. Bond, S. Peace, F. Dittmann-Kohli & G. Westerhoff (Eds.), *Ageing in society* (pp. 268–295). London, England: Sage.

Estes, C. L. (2001). *Social policy and aging: A critical perspective*. London, England: Sage.

European Union. (2012). European year of active ageing & intergenerational solidarity 2012. Retrieved May 8, 2017, from www.age-platform.eu/images/stories/EY2012_Campaign.pdf

Featherstone, M., & Hepworth, M. (1989). Ageing and old age: Reflections on the postmodern life course. In B. Bytheway, T. Keil, P. Allatt & A. Bryman (Eds.), *Becoming and being old: Sociological approaches to later life* (pp. 143–157). London, England: Sage.

Foucault, M. (1976/1981). *Discipline and punish*. London, England: Penguin Books.

Fries, J. F. (1980). Aging, natural death, and the compression of morbidity. *New England Journal of Medicine, 303*(3), 130.

Gilleard, C., & Higgs, P. (2005). Contexts of ageing: Class, cohort and community. Cambridge, UK: Polity Press.

International Labour Organization. (2015). *World social protection report 2014/15: Building economic recovery, inclusive development and social justice*. Geneva, Switzerland: Author.

Irwin, S. (1998). Age, generation and inequality. *British Journal of Sociology, 49*, 305–310.

Jung, C. G. (1932/1967). *Collected works* (Vol. 7). London, England: Routledge.

Kohli, M. (2005). Generational changes and generational equity. In Malcolm L. Johnson (ed.), *The Cambridge Handbook of Age and Ageing* (pp. 518–526). Cambridge: Cambridge University Press.

Martinson, M., & Halpern, J. (2011). Ethical implications of the promotion of elder volunteerism: A critical perspective. *Journal of Aging Studies, 25*(4), 427–435.

Metz, D., & Underwood, M. (2005). *Older richer fitter: Identifying the customer needs of Britain's ageing population*. London, England: Age Concern Books.

Moody, H. R. (2001). Productive aging and the ideology of old age. In N. Morrow-Howell, J. Hinterlong & M. Sherraden (Eds.), *Productive aging: Concepts and challenges* (pp. 175–196). Baltimore, MD: Johns Hopkins University Press.

Moulaert, T., & Biggs, S. (2013). International and European policy on work and retirement: Reinventing critical perspectives on active ageing and mature subjectivity. *Human Relations, 66*(1), 23–43.

Olshansky, J. (2007, July). *Securing the longevity dividend*. Paper presented at the Securing the Longevity Dividend: Building the Campaign for Anti-Aging Science, Chicago, USA.

Phillipson, C. (1998). *Reconstructing old age: New agendas in social theory and practice*. London, England: Sage.

Phillipson, C. (2012). Globalisation, economic recession and social exclusion: Policy challenges and responses. In T. Scharf & N. Keating (Eds.), *From exclusion to inclusion in old age: A global challenge* (pp. 17–32). Bristol, England: Policy Press.

Piketty, T., (2014). *Capital in the twenty-first century: The dynamics of inequality, wealth, and growth*. Cambridge, MA: The Belknap Press of Harvard University Press.

Rowe, J. W., & Kahn, R. L. (1987). Human aging: Usual and successful. *Science, 237*, 143–150.

Standing, G. (2011). *The precariat: The new dangerous class*. New York, NY: Bloomsbury Academic.

Tornstam, L. (2005). *Gerotranscendence: A developmental theory of positive aging*. New York, NY: Springer Publishing Company.

United Nations. (1982). *Vienna international plan of action on aging*. Report of the world assembly on aging. Retrieved from www.un.org/esa/socdev/ageing/documents/Resources/VIPEE-English.pdf

United Nations. (2002). *Madrid international plan of action on aging.* New York, NY: Author.

United Nations. (2016). *World population prospects: The 2010 revision.* New York, NY: Author.

van Dyk, S. (2014). The appraisal of difference: Critical gerontology and the active ageing paradigm. *Journal of Aging Studies, 31,* 93–103.

Walker, A. (2009). Commentary: The emergence and application of active aging in Europe. *Journal of Aging & Social Policy, 21,* 75–93.

World Health Organization. (2002). *Active ageing: A policy framework.* Second World Assembly on Aging. Madrid, Spain: Author.

World Health Organization. (2007). *Age-friendly cities: A checklist.* Geneva, Switzerland: Author.

2   Interrogating personal and intergenerational ageing

Key themes

- How an ageing identity negotiates personal and social priorities
- Generational intelligence as a means of understanding other age groups
- Resolving tensions between continuity and change
- Examining the importance of positive discontinuity and positive otherness
- Distinguishing between within-age and between-age thinking
- Adopting a present-centred or lifetime-centred approach

Negotiating generational intelligence, identity management and narrative

If we are to more easily understand how the personal and the social dimensions of adult ageing can be brought together and therefore negotiate ageing identities and relationships, a number of issues need to be drawn into sharper focus. These centre around the changing lifecourse as an important factor in being able to make judgements between the options that society presents, particularly as they affect ways of living a long life and intergenerational relationships. Once one accepts that the adult lifecourse consists of different phases, each with its own set of tasks and priorities, then the question of how to make connections between these different phases and the people who inhabit them becomes visible.

A key element in the process of making links between different life priorities has been called generational intelligence. It charts the degree to which people recognise generational differences, the consequences of locating or ignoring distinctive age-based life phases, and the possibilities for negotiation between distinctive generational groups. Key here is the idea that individuals vary in the degree of generational intelligence they can deploy, depending upon the context in which they encounter other age groups and perceive themselves as holding particular age-based identities.

In the first part of this chapter, generational intelligence will be briefly described. Then concepts that may be useful in interrogating some of the 'solutions' to the question of age identity and intergenerational relationships will be explored. These concepts follow from generational intelligence as a critical tool and include positive discontinuity in lifecourse development as a motor for change, positive otherness as it exists between generational groups, the question of whether narratives around ageing reflect 'within-age' or 'between-age' thinking, and whether a present-centred or lifecourse-centred perspective is adopted.

As part of this exploration, the way that people manage their age-based identities will be examined in more detail, exploring the processes by which narratives might skew how identity is expressed in age-sensitive interaction. It is argued that dominant narratives, such as those associated with work, belief, bodily ageing and family relations will influence the possibilities for protecting the ageing self and connecting with others. The balance achieved between generational intelligence, continuity, and change will affect how persons and societies adapt to the living of a long life. It constitutes an attempt to make sense of the options made available by social and cultural realities, which in various combinations can be accepted or resisted or provoke alternatives.

Lifecourse specificity and generational intelligence

Lifecourse change and its implications for ageing, intergenerational relations, and social policy is a key element of the approach explored in this book. They are the special focus of this inquiry as an alternative way of understanding the most powerful narratives of the day. And while there are many ways of examining identity, such as through gender, ethnicity and sexual orientation, the principle focus here will be on the personal and social influence of age and adult ageing.

Examining changes across the lifecourse, through childhood to adolescence, the first period of adulthood, midlife and late life, right into deep old age, forms a material base on which to judge the value of policies and social expectations that attempt to shape the way we live our lives. They are, barring individual accidents, illnesses and wider environmental and political disasters, a pathway through which most people, most of the time can expect to travel. They are rooted in biological change but subject to personal and social interpretation. Even with a longer life span, the same phases are passed through, even though they can be stretched to fit a longer time period. Examples here may be the socially determined expectations on how long one stays in education or an increase in healthy lifestyles that pushes back the age of infirmity. This stretching of the lifecourse is subject to a complex interconnection of biological, psychological and social factors, but nevertheless the lifecourse itself supplies a material platform and an anchor through which to locate human experience.

When compared to the shifting sands of that other form of material base, economics, a lifecourse-based approach supplies something that is less uneven and less subject to radical shifts of fortune. It is, in other words, a common and relatively stable experience that nearly all human beings can use as a way of negotiating their changing identities. For most individuals the assumption that people of different ages bring different skills, priorities and therefore contributions to the table is so obvious that it sounds a little mad to have to state it. Unfortunately the narratives underlying a number of contemporary policies on ageing appear to eclipse this fundamental source of diversity.

An important element in the journey towards discovering a long life's purpose and how one relates to others with an awareness of age is encompassed by generational intelligence (Biggs & Lowenstein, 2011, Biggs, Haapala & Lowenstein, 2011). Generational intelligence picks up on an understanding that different phases of life contain different priorities. The challenges facing an adolescent searching for an adult identity and the youthful adult starting a career and seeking a serious partner, plus the challenges of midlife and older age each hold a distinctive set of developmental tasks (Erikson, 1989), which while they are not exclusive to those stages set up a series of challenges that require resolution in a particular way. If different age groups contain different priorities, it is argued by generational intelligence, then that how to understand the age-other becomes a question that cannot be taken for granted and has to be resolved.

Generational intelligence, starting with the transition between what Jung (1932/1967) had called the first and second halves of life, explores the consequences that follow once lifecourse differences take shape in adulthood (see Biggs, 1999). It poses the question: How far is it possible to put yourself into the shoes of someone of a different age group? As such, it highlights tension between age-specific life tasks and intergenerational connection as it can no longer be assumed that all adults have the same orientation and understandings of how that might be resolved. For once one has recognised oneself as part of a specific age group or generation, then one has separated oneself off from other age groups and needs to return to them in some way without losing this new awareness of self and of a distinctive other. Generational intelligence highlights the importance of the degree to which one becomes conscious of self as part of a generation or age group, the relative ability to put yourself in the position of other generations and the relative ability to then negotiate between generational positions.

Any person or set of social arrangements can contain high or low degrees of generational intelligence. Low intelligence is evidenced by a lack of capacity for recognising others beyond one's own needs and perspective, and high generational intelligence shows an ability to empathise with an alternative life position and build complementary relations between oneself and others. Getting to generational intelligence includes four steps, which are explored by Biggs, Haapala and Lowenstein (2011). These include recognising that one is part of a generation or age group, identifying distinctive features of different ages and generations, taking a value stance towards similarities and differences that emerge and finally acting on the basis of these sources of distinction. A high degree of generational intelligence, it is argued, would be evidenced by an ability to recognise age-based distinctiveness and overlaps, plus agreement on mutually acceptable ways forward. If people are to act in a manner that requires negotiation between age groups, then generational intelligence needs to be high.

An understanding of changing lifecourse priorities and encounters between different age groups or generations introduces a number of phenomena, which may help us tackle our two questions of new cultural adaptations and purposes provoked by population ageing.

Continuity and change

A set of assumptions that come into tension as a result of this psychosocial analysis of the lifecourse are those between sameness and changes to identity, sometimes called continuity versus discontinuity. Traditionally, within social gerontology, it has been assumed that older adults wish to stay the same, that is, to keep the identity that they have developed in previous periods of their lives, and that a significant amount of energy is used in maintaining that situation. Continuity theory was first proposed by Robert Atchley in 1989. 'People,' he said, 'are predisposed and motivated towards inner psychological continuity as well as outward continuity of social behaviour and circumstances' (1989: 24), and as such, the theory assumes that ageing persons have the need and the tendency to maintain the same habits and perspectives that they developed over their lifecourse to date. And while recognising ageing as an interaction between biological, psychological and social changes, continuity theory emphasises the effort people put into preserving pre-existing habits, preferences and lifestyles. Ageing is seen as a struggle for stability in the face of various forms of transience, and because of this, people seek out situations that confirm their existing identities and their current social habits (Atchley, 2009). The struggle with social forces, such as ageism, would then be around fending off threats to carrying on in the same way as before.

A problem for continuity is that, as the midlife counselling psychologist Dan McAdams (1993) has pointed out, uncertainties around social expectations on ageing mean that as 'our world can no longer tell us who we are and how we should live, we must figure it out on our own' (1993). When this is added to the Jungian (1932/1967) insight that the dynamic of the adult lifecourse leads to dissatisfaction with social conformity as 'first half of life' achievements in work, family building and social standing give way to yearning for new 'second half' goals, assumptions about continuity begin to unravel. Priorities rooted in the lifecourse can change and even if they are resisted, still pose a significant new dynamic for personal identity. Maintaining continuity then becomes a rear-guard strategy to preserve some kind of pre-existing certainty in a changing environment, rather than embracing the potential released by what Jung call individuation.

Continuity, seen from the perspective of generational intelligence, reinforces an unwillingness to encounter distinctiveness based on age and highlights the latter's focus on discontinuity and changing priorities between different life phases. While we generally want to be seen as continuous in the sense of holding consistent values and 'in being the same person' over time, generational difference means that we also need to generate different priorities depending upon where we are in the lifecourse.

To develop a sense of a continuous self that can adapt to changing priorities requires a series of critical developments in the way we think about the purpose and contribution of a long life. First of these would be becoming aware of oneself as a member of a particular age group or generation. If priorities differ between ages, then sameness becomes a less effective assumptive reality to inhabit. This gives rise to a second question for identity, how if ages are different, does one come to terms with individuals and groups of other age groups. Does one attempt to erase difference, to compete against the age-other, or to find consensus between generational groups? And finally how is one to act while being mindful of inter-generational space and its multiple agendas?

A 'more of the same' approach is evident in continuity theory and also in productive ageing approaches (Morrow-Howell, Hinterlong & Sherraden, 2001), and to a degree in medical definitions of functional age (WHO, 2002), however, a number of writers have emphasised the discontinuous qualities of long-lived experience. The notion of adaptation implies that there is a qualitative as well as a quantitative distinction to be made as the different generations become more equal in demographic size. There is emerging evidence that while individuals desire continuity of identity, this does not preclude discontinuity of age-related life priorities and the negotiation of a set of changing existential tasks that face adults as they grow older (Tornstam, 2005; Dittman-Kohli & Joop, 2007). These tasks include taking into account finitude (that we will eventually die and that this is getting closer), limitation (on the time left to do things, make one's peace with others and achieve cherished goals) and integration (to express previously suppressed parts of oneself and gain some sense of oneself and one's life as a whole). A focus on a discontinuity of psychosocial priorities across the adult lifecourse also raises the issue of the degree to which intergenerational agendas overlap and the idea that a solution to generational solidarity may lie less on causing generational rivalry over the same territory but in developing complementary roles and relationships (Biggs, 2014).

Unthought knowns and positive discontinuity

Simone De Beauvoir, in her seminal book, *La Viellesse* (1970), translated as 'Old Age' in the UK and in the United States as 'Coming of Age' observed 'When we are grown-up, we hardly think about our age any more: we feel the notion doesn't apply to us, we are reaching out towards the future gliding on imperceptible from day to day, from year to year'. Old age is particularly difficult to assume because we have always regarded it as a foreign species: 'Can I have become a different being while I still remain myself?' (DeBeauvoir, 1970: 315).

One of the problems in identifying themes that go against the stream is that there may be little explicit recognition of them, particularly in the public sphere. They are often tacitly acknowledged but obscured by forms of identity management and masquerades that seek to protect their underlying processes. It is no accident that some of the key proponents of discontinuous identities in mid- and later life, have been psychotherapists, whose job it has been to examine the relationship between the hidden and the surfaces of identity (Jung, 1931; Erikson, 1989; Vaillant, 2002; Bollas, 2012; Montero et al., 2012). Ageing itself, in so far as everybody wants a long life but no one wants to grow old appeared to be, what Bollas (1987) has called, an 'unthought known'. In other words, adult ageing seems to bring a series of tacit assumptions into play and, with higher degrees of generational intelligence, into consciousness, which, while most people most of the time do not give them voice, shape personal experience. At a deep level, they are known, yet at a surface level, their presence is either avoided or denied. It raises the possibility that ageing is in some way recognised by individuals, but they are often unable to think about it. Ageing becomes something that one 'knows about' but does not 'think about', except as a thing without content, to be avoided through anti-ageing supplements and cosmetics. Thinking about ageing, in the everyday run of things, may rarely go beyond surface appearances, failing to explore what it signals to the self. It is only when the unthought travels into the territory of the thinkable that adaptation, both cultural and personal, can begin to take shape.

Paying attention to alternatives to lifecourse continuity as more of the same, places discontinuity in a more positive light. In psychotherapy, it has been noted (Freud, 1909/1962; Jung, 1931/1967; Yalom, 1980) that resistance to change can be most vigorous just before that change is about to happen, an observation that Jung and his followers (Samuels et al., 1986) identify with the midlife transition from the first to the second half of adult life. It indicates that resistance to a change in life's purpose may itself be part of a process of incipient transformation. It is here that positive discontinuity becomes interesting. It is another word for change and development over time. In terms of ageing, permitting positive discontinuity to emerge would involve allowing the unthought to become known and the clinging to continuity to be overcome.

Positive discontinuity refers to the advantages that occur once age-related change is acknowledged rather than feared. It allows the social actor to engage with alternatives to dominant interpretations of what it means to grow old and one's stance towards that process. A recognition of discontinuity also allows one to stand back and see the other more clearly as a distinct entity, based on age. Once these forms of discontinuity are available to conscious scrutiny, overlaps and differences in perspective can be more easily understood. Positive discontinuity, then, opens the possibility of being attentive to the implications of not being the same, both personally over time and between people of different age groups. Without it, maturity, as the process of progressive development associated with growing older, would be harder to recognise and achieve as would be personal awareness of one's own position vis-à-vis others. Without an understanding of the positive implications of discontinuity of age identity, it would be much more likely that overlap is misrecognised as similarity and change identified as being negative in itself. With positive discontinuity, we not only become different whilst remaining ourselves; we become more closely attuned to the distinctiveness of others.

Recognising positive discontinuity, the awareness of change provoked by increased generational intelligence, would allow adaptation to take place in both the personal and public spheres. However, ensuring that this can take place would require a public debate on ageing that values age-related change and distinctiveness between generations.

Hidden, surface and narrative impact

The promise of positive discontinuity raises the question of how to manage an age-based identity in a world where there are competing narratives on age and generation. How do the processes of managing an ageing identity adapt to changed circumstances, inversions of expectation, the presentation of legitimising narratives and evolving lifecourse priorities?

Understanding how an ageing identity is managed has often relied on exploring the tension between hidden and surface elements of identity, whether through a 'mask of ageing' (Hepworth, 2004), masquerade (Woodward, 1991; Butler, 2012) or persona and masque (Biggs, 1999, 2004). Masking, then, is a way of thinking about how we engage with the social world that relies upon the analogy of performance. The mask and the performance change, depending upon the context a person is in and the particular demands for self-presentation that the actor is under. As certain identities are performed, the aim is usually to best find a balance between our inner thoughts, feelings and beliefs and external pressures, such as requirements to conform to certain predetermined stereotypes and roles.

The mask, or masque, forms the boundary between personal and social worlds. The distinction between a persona or social mask and a masque is important in so far as the masque reaches beyond bodily appearance or conformity with fixed social categories to include the deployment of any number of props, attributes and social routines. Different elements in a masque, as they reflect a changing dynamic between hidden and surface elements of identity, may be more fixed or fluid than others, depending upon the different periods of life being lived through and the demands of any one narrative context. The masque can include the 'raw material' of the ageing body; the use of cosmetics, clothing, posture, diet and exercise; non-verbal behaviour; social skills; specific contexts and other props to create a desired effect.

Seeing ageing as a narrative sets up a tension between the internal world of the imagination, the external world of the immediate environment, and the mask itself, which forms the bridge between the two. In midlife, tensions may emerge between narratives of a youthful persona and the pressure to adapt to a mature identity (Biggs et al., 2007). Jung (1932/1967) saw the persona as an impediment to self-actualisation and progression into the next life phase that became particularly acute in midlife, while Goffman (1963) has emphasised the protective qualities of performance. An increased awareness of the role of social ageism makes it clear that pressure to conform does not end with midlife. And while Jung has put his finger on an essential truth – that social conformity can limit psychosocial development and needs to be confronted if continued personal development is to take place – he did not recognise the continuing role of ageism as a limiting narrative factor.

Under such conditions, dominant narratives form the ground against which an ageing identity is protected and influences the possibilities for connecting to the social world. In the case of adult ageing, this would include the need to protect new potential and self-awareness and the validity of preceding experience from-age related expectation and threat. But also to make connections with others in ways that are both visible and interpersonally valid to age peers and to other age groups and generations.

The relationship between inner and outer realities and masquerade is best seen as a process rather than a set of contents. The contents, what is hidden and what is surface, would, according to this perspective, change depending upon the social and historical circumstances ageing adults find themselves in. For example, if stereotyping, in the form of narrative, demands that the older adult withdraw from society and asserts that he or she has no active contribution to make and anyway older people are seen as a homogeneous group without the capacity for individual eccentricity, then life forces that draw the individual towards increased individuation, of becoming more oneself and expressing hitherto suppressed capabilities, will themselves be suppressed, although they might still live an undercover existence. If the expectation is that to earn a place in society, the older adult will need to be active, productive and socially engaged, then alternative forms of self-expression, which might include, spirituality, reflection, and what Tornstam (2005) refers to as 'positive solitude' may find themselves hidden. In a society that expects spiritual development in later life, material routes to fulfilment may be forced undercover and vice versa. There may be multiple narratives at work, but they cannot all be performed at once, and the salience of one presupposes the submersion, or attempted submersion, of other elements of identity. The balance between hidden and surface would vary depending upon whether one was at work, with one's family, engaging in spiritual development, or attending health services. It draws attention to the degree to which others are seen as 'other' and the circumstances in which othering is necessary in order to make genuine contact with someone who is different. Positive discontinuity would involve negotiating the relationship both between changing life priorities, self and other and consciousness of what is recognised and what has been suppressed.

Age-otherness and positive othering

An age-other, according to Biggs and Lowenstein (2011) is

> someone who is constructed as being of a different group to oneself, based on age. Age-otherness may include aspects of lifecourse and family position and cohort identity. Whether an individual is seen as being 'other' will be affected by the interaction of these elements of generational identity.
>
> (2011: xii)

Identifying another person as being of a different age, an age-other, is not necessarily a quantifiable difference, but is rather phenomenologically real in the sense that a difference is perceived to exist by one or both of the actors involved. Under optimal conditions, persons who identify as being of different age groups would be able to put themselves in the position of the age-other. Biggs and Lowenstein (2011) also distinguish between 'simple' and 'complex' thinking, the latter being more demanding as it requires that the participants do not assume that the other holds similar attitudes and beliefs to themselves.

In this context, negotiation implies that there is a qualitative as well as a quantitative distinction to be made as different generations become more equal in size. And, rather than attempting an erasure of any transition in life priorities, future directions should ensure recognition of the special qualities that a long life brings with it. The tension here is principally to do the boundaries that are set around age-otherness. How does one see a person or group as different to oneself in terms of age categories and to what degree is that difference rooted in the actual qualities of the other?

The process of 'othering' refers to seeing another person as different to the self and is most commonly associated with forms of age prejudice. As Phillips, Ajrouch & Hillcoat-Nallétamby (2010) have pointed out:

> Every individual has the potential to experience discrimination or prejudice based on their age if they live long enough. It produces an 'othering' effect that lumps all those considered old into a category defined, first, as different and, secondly as inferior. More importantly, it suggests that all old people are alike, hence obscuring differences that exist among and between older persons.
>
> (Phillips et al., 2010: 21)

The psychosocial processes underlying this form of negative othering rely upon the projection of undesirable parts of the self onto others so that they can then safely be attacked and disparaged. It is a form of pushing away in order to distance oneself from negative associations and attributes. As part of this process, only parts that conform to negative difference are recognised and the possibility of a more comprehensive engagement is lost. It then becomes possible to treat the other as not fully human and avoid the difficult emotions that would arise in so doing. So, while projection seems to create a recognition of difference, it is only an absorption of the age-other into a pre-existing set of stereotypes. In terms of age, this might include blaming the old for being dependent or vulnerable, so as to preserve the phantasy of the invulnerability of the self (Dartington, 2013). It may justify the ascription of older retirees as being lazy or greedy, whilst secretly desiring a break from the demands of a stressful and overdemanding workplace. It permits an envious attack on the thing that is not me – who become demonised as an economic burden, a bed blocker or as someone who should get out of the way and give his or her job to a younger individual. Negative othering also allows a replacement of the actual attributes and desires of the other by those of a dominant narrative or age group. This process has been elaborated by Biggs (2004), calling it 'The colonization of the goals, aims, priorities and agendas of one age-group by another. This may be consciously done for reasons of political and economic expediency, or unknowingly as if these priorities are simply commonsense' (2004: 103).

Members of a dominant age group or generation are thereby enabled to unthinkingly assume that their perceptions are universally valid. Negative othering becomes an unthought known of the intergenerational encounter, where age dominance takes superiority for granted and is reflected as part of the equation that one's own group's reality can legitimately override alternative positions.

There is a way, however, that otherness based on age fulfils a positive function. This emerges through a recognition that in order to see the other more fully, it is necessary to separate self and other out in the mind's eye, in order to return with refreshed insight (Faimberg, 2005; Biggs & Lowenstein, 2011). The distinctive identities of others based on age can then be identified and a more genuine form of relationship can potentially emerge. Rather than a process of rejection, this would ultimately become a process of connection as the other person is approached as someone with his or her own characteristics, projects and idioms. By separating out the perspectives of self and other, rather than assuming that they are both the same, an individual becomes aware of his or her own particular identity and achieves a newfound freedom of expression. This allows a critical reflective space to emerge in which the boundaries between oneself and others become more clearly negotiated. The outcome would be that one can now see the other person as distinctive, and it becomes possible to engage in genuine dialogue. This is important in terms of age, in so far as it allows someone to be more aware of their own generational perspective and to respect rather than ignore alternative positions.

Positive othering constitutes a willingness to consider distinctiveness based on adult age, even if these do not correspond with the dominant group's interests and world view. Once the respective positons of the protagonists are recognised and given voice, it is then possible to begin a process of realistic understanding, based on the actual rather than assumed positions of the age-other. It allows the complementary nature of relationships to emerge.

Within- and between-age thinking

The preceding discussion on generational intelligence, positive discontinuity and othering provokes us to distinguish between debates, policies and narratives that engage in 'within-age' and 'between-age' thinking. Where discontinuity and othering examine the boundaries between interior and exterior realities and how identities, individuals and groups are included or pushed away, within- and between-age thinking is focussed on where boundaries are drawn around debates and how priorities for action are identified. It refers to where horizons are set in the process of making a phenomenon manageable and as such provides a means of examining what is included and what is left out. This is an important distinction to make if we are to begin to understand how the purpose of a long life and the relations between generations and age groups are played out in services and in policy debates.

'Within-age thinking' is principally concerned with working out processes, projects and implications that are contained through a consideration of a single defined age or generational group. As such, the issues under consideration are part of a closed system, and boundaries have been drawn around the debate that exclude alternative perspectives or other groups.

'Between-age thinking' is concerned with the interaction between groups defined by age or generational difference. It is therefore a more open system than within-age thinking, although boundaries are still drawn around what constitutes a group and which groups are included.

So within-age thinking might concentrate on a policy response to the problems of a particular age group in itself. Between-age thinking would focus on the connection between one age group and another. And while a distinction between within- and between-age thinking may often be a matter of degree, certain policy discourses will consider an age group principally in isolation and another might look at it intergenerationally.

Each has advantages and disadvantages, in so far as examining the circumstances of a particular age group allows their specific qualities, contents and processes to be considered with minimum contamination by other perspectives. However, meaning is also generated between individuals and groups, and the conduct of one group or debate about that group rarely stands in isolation – the no-one-is-an-island effect. Debate on which is best crops up in a variety of places, for example on whether there should be specialist geriatric services or whether they should be part and parcel of general adult care, whether specific elder protection services are better than generic adult protection, or whether we need a specific convention on the rights of older people. It also raises the tricky question of how intergenerational dilemmas should be resolved.

For current purposes, a distinction between with- and between-age thinking allows insight into whether a debate is considering one generational position or the interaction between positions. The weight given to each would be a matter of degree depending upon focus and context, and different parts of a debate may be concentrated on particular forms of thinking. It could be argued, for example, that debates on older workers at the beginning of the 21st century conceived work as a between-age problem (who should be working and for how long), generating within-age thinking (early or later retirement, age-friendly workplaces, age-targeted recruitment and retention policies). Whereas pension policy has been seen as addressing a within-age problem (support to older adults), stimulating between-age thinking (generational transfers, rebalancing or solidarity). The degree to which within- and between-age thinking takes place shapes the way social issues are addressed and responded to.

Present-centredness and lifetime-centredness

Another form of boundary setting can be seen between present-centred and lifetime-centred thinking. Here, distinctions are made on a temporal basis with the former focussing on the here and now and the latter placing events in a longitudinal context. Generational intelligence in this context involves an enhanced sensitivity to thinking about relationships marked by time. Lifetime thinking could be thought of as long term and strategic, while present-centred thinking is short term and tactical.

Present-centred thinking would emphasise the process of current relations and reflects an absorption in everyday experience. As such, it has a tendency to characterise the passage of time as a process that the social actor is not consciously aware of, giving life an ageless quality. It reflects de Beauvoir's notion of ageing 'not applying to us'. Things occur in a continuous present, which can be forward looking but without necessarily engaging with temporal context and longer historical perspectives. The time horizon is sometimes no longer than days, with sameness, repetition and recycling taking priority. Present-centred thinking is marked by an interpretation of experience as it is absorbed in the everyday. Unevenness is problematic. In one sense, present-centredness is tremendously important. It is the point of our current and immediate engagement with the world. Over time, things come and go, but as temporal creatures, we are forever living in the present.

Lifetime-centred thinking would emphasise change within a lifecourse horizon, a long duration, beyond immediate experience, and incorporates a sense of past, present and future. Lifetime is marked by rhythms or waves that play themselves out over years rather than days. An awareness of lifetime produces a distinctive attitude to transience, to time and its passage, that places particular experiences as representing one point in an evolutionary process. Lifetime thinking is marked by a consciousness of distinctive periods of experience and engagement in context, both sequential and rhythmic. At any one time, one is thereby attuned to a particular set of lifetime priorities, which, at its best, can generate an intelligence of long temporal rhythms and age-specific priorities. The importance of lifetime thinking lies in its ability to see interconnection and cumulative effects. While things may come and go, their consequences can stay with us and determine the futures we lead.

Viewed from a lifetime perspective, the unfairness of *present-centred thinking*, as a yardstick for social value, lies in the evacuation of the past. When we think about our own pensions, for example, many of us think longitudinally. It's an investment, a contract between ourselves and the state over a long period of time. Thinking cross-sectionally, as many policy makers do, it's about money coming in and going out during one financial year. The combination of these two perspectives raises questions of trust that what is offered now will be present in the future.

Present-centredness can contribute to an amnesia of the effort that older generations had contributed. And when lifetime-centredness is recognised, it can easily be seen as 'living in the past', while it is actually a form of 'living with the past' (Biggs, 1999). Living with rather than avoiding the past is a key element in the healing process of the psychotherapies and probably the greatest insight of Freudian analysis (Freud, 1909/1962). It stops us repeating our mistakes and sets the scene for novel directions. The seductive conceit that we are ageless, non-transient beings, is however a key feature of contemporary life. Baars (2012) points to the ageless person being synonymous with a 'normal vigorous adulthood', with adult ageing then categorised as 'an abnormal process'. Deviation from present-centredness becomes an unwelcome reminder of vulnerability and interdependence. He states,

> Through influential but illusive images of youth, *the vulnerability* inherent in life is pushed out of sight, evoking an abstract image of a 'normal' world that knows only happiness, health and selfconfident winners . . . a 'normal' vigourous adulthood, which can be subjected to protracted stress without any problem.
>
> (202).

At a psychosocial level, it is known that we all will grow old, barring external shocks or the roll of the genetic dice. But in everyday consciousness, the fact is often suppressed, even though, in contrast to other forms of social identity, such as gender or ethnicity, we are more likely to enter that state ourselves, becoming the age-other over time. In an everyday sense, the promise of personal ageing is rarely thought about beyond the surfaces of immediate narrative content. Lifetime-centredness provides an antidote.

The ways that dominant narratives shape our expectations of ageing and possibilities for personal expression is a key component of the rest of this book. Narratives on ageing and generational relations, concerning the value of work, spirituality, the body and family will be taken in turn to see how ageing has been negotiated. Positive discontinuity and otherness, within- and between-age thinking and present- and lifetime-centredness, each in different ways, elaborate the power of a generationally intelligent perspective. They provide us with tools that can be used to make sense of narratives on ageing that swarm around us as we encounter ageing in self and others. And it is to those debates that we will now turn.

References

Atchley, R. C. (1989). A continuity theory of normal aging. *The Gerontologist, 29*(2), 183–190.

Atchley, R. C. (2009). *Spirituality and aging.* Baltimore, MD: Johns Hopkins University Press.

Baars, J. (2012). *Aging and the art of living.* Baltimore, MD: Johns Hopkins University Press.

Biggs, S. (1999). *The mature imagination: Dynamics of identity in midlife and beyond.* Buckingham, England: Open University Press.

Biggs, S. (2004). Age, gender, narratives, and masquerades. *Journal of Aging Studies, 18*(1), 45–58.

Biggs, S. (2014). Adapting to an ageing society, the need for cultural change. *Policy Quarterly, 10*(3), 12–17.

Biggs, S., Haapala, I., & Lowenstein, A. (2011). Exploring generational intelligence as a model for examining the process of intergenerational relationships. *Ageing and Society, 31*(7), 1107–1124.

Biggs, S., & Lowenstein, A. (2011). *Generational intelligence: A critical approach to age relations.* New York, NY: Routledge.

Biggs, S., Phillipson, C., Leach, R., & Money, A. M. (2007). The mature imagination and consumption strategies: Age & generation in the development of a United Kingdom baby boomer identity. *International Journal of Ageing and Later Life, 2*(2), 31–59.

Bollas, C. (1987). *The shadow of the object.* London, England: Free Association Books.

Bollas, C. (1992). *Being a character: Psychoanalysis and self-experience.* London, England: Free Association Books.

Bollas, C. (2012). Interview with Christopher Bollas. In G. J. Montero, A. M. C. de Montero, & L. S. de Vogelfanger (Eds.), *Updating midlife: Psychoanalytic perspectives.* London: Karnac Books.

Butler, J. (2012). *Subjects of desire: Hegelian reflections in twentieth-century France.* New York, NY: Columbia University Press.

Dartington, T. (2013). Meeting the needs of vulnerable patients. *Nursing Management, 19*(9), 12–12.

DeBeauvoir, S. (1970). *Old age*. London, England: Weidenfeld and Nicolson.

Dittman-Kohli, F., & Joop, D. (2007). Self and life management. In J. Bond, S. Peace, F. Dittmann-Kohli & G. Westerhoff (Eds.), *Ageing in society* (pp. 268–295). London, England: Sage.

Erikson, E. H. (1989). *The life cycle completed*. New York, NY: W.W. Norton & Company.

Faimberg, H. (2005). *The telescoping of generations: Listening to the narcissistic links between generations*. London, England: Routledge.

Freud, S. (1909/1962). *Two short accounts of psychoanalysis*. London, England: Penguin Books.

Goffman, E. (1963). *Behavior in public places*. New York, NY: Free Press.

Hepworth, M. (2004). Embodied agency, decline and the mask of ageing. In E. Tulle (Ed.), *Old age and agency* (pp. 125–136). New York, NY: Nova.

Jung, C. G. (1931). *The aims of psychotherapy*. London, England: Routledge.

Jung, C. G. (1931/1967). *Collected works* (Vol. 9). London, England: Routledge.

Jung, C. G. (1932/1967). *Collected works* (Vol. 7). London, England: Routledge.

Jung, C. G. (1933). *Modern man in search of a soul*. London, England: Kegan Paul Trench Trubner, (1955 ed. Harvest Books ISBN 0-15-661206-2).

McAdams, D. P. (1993). *The stories we live by: Personal myths and the making of the self*. New York, NY: Guilford Press.

Montero, G. J., de Montero, A. M. C., & de Vogelfanger, L. S. (2012). *Updating midlife: Psychoanalytic perspectives*. London, England: Karnac Books.

Morrow-Howell, N., Hinterlong, J., & Sherraden, M. (Eds.). (2001). *Productive aging: Concepts and challenges*. Baltimore, MD: Johns Hopkins University Press.

Phillips, J. E., Ajrouch, K. J., & Hillcoat-Nallétamby, S. (2010). *Key concepts in social gerontology*. Los Angeles, CA: Sage.

Samuels, A., Shorter, B., & Plaut, F. (1986). *A critical dictionary of jungian analysis*. London, England: Routledge and Kagan-Paul.

Tornstam, L. (2005). *Gerotranscendence: A developmental theory of positive aging*. New York, NY: Springer Publishing Company.

Vaillant, G. E. (2002). *Aging well*. Boston, MA: Little, Brown and Company.

Woodward, K. (1991). *Aging and its discontents: Freud and other fictions*. Bloomington, IN: Indiana University Press.

World Health Organization. (2002). *Active ageing: A policy framework*. Second World Assembly on Aging. Madrid, Spain: Author.

Yalom, I. D. (1980). *Existential psychotherapy*. New York, NY: Basic Books.

3   Work to the rescue?

Key themes

- Work as the accepted policy solution to a long life
- Older and younger workers may be better at different things
- Lifetime and immediate experience of working life both influence decisions to stay or leave work
- Alternative sources of income influence decisions to work or retire
- Attitudes to personal ageing influence attitudes to continued working or stopping work
- A focus on productivism and continuity can eclipse generational distinctiveness

Work policy appears to adopt a within-age and present-centred narrative. The shift towards work in later life

At the beginning of the 21st century, public debate on ageing shifted. Prior to that time, much had been made of the increasing dependency, both bodily and economic, that accompanies growing older. Moving from the 20th to the 21st, the focus was first on capitalising on the increased spending power of 'active agers' and the filling out of a 'third age,' which came between working life and the fourth age of decline, with consumer activity and then challenging compulsory exclusions from working life itself. During the global economic recession of the twenty-teens, however, a trend to encourage older working as a human rights issue mutated into a compulsion to work longer fuelled mainly by the erosion of pension eligibility. In some countries, this was accompanied by an attempt to set one generation against another (see Chapter 10), with work and the cost of pensions as the instruments of choice. Whatever one might think of these trends, the relationship between work and adult ageing emerges as a laboratory for the degree to which a long life is flexible at the hands of social policy.

An important consequence of these shifts has been that new questions have begun to arise that place ageing as a key component of political and public discourse. Should older workers be encouraged to stay longer in employment? Should they be forced to take work? Are there differences between younger and older workers in their attitude to working life? Is work the right thing to fill the extra years of longevity? And what sort of social capital does a long life bring with it (Biggs, Carstensen & Hogan, 2012)? The debate has been heated. It has led to a serious critical debate within social gerontology as to whether extending working life is an answer to social ageism or simply ageism in a different form (van Dyk, 2014)? It is a debate that is particularly pointed because, on the one hand, many older adults have accrued social capital that could be put to good use and, on the other, continued work until one is no longer capable would be exploitative and ignorant of the changing lifecourse.

From its first significant mention by the Organisation for Economic Cooperation and Development (OECD) (1988b) and the World Bank in 1994, population ageing has, as a consequence of its association with employment, migrated from the margins to the centre of contemporary social policy. Here, ageing has most often been characterised as an exterior threat; indeed, few of the veterans of 1968 would have thought that this was the way that they would eventually pose a challenge to the capitalist system. In this context, the work of the World Bank (1994) and the OECD (2006) plus the policy statements of numerous nation-states (see USA, 1997; European Union, 2012; Commonwealth of Australia, 2015; UK, 2017) show an emerging international policy consensus. This consensus marks a shift away from a holistic approach to the inclusion of older adults to one that focusses almost entirely on work as the means of filling the additional years of a long life. This view appears to have become increasingly entrenched following the global financial crisis. It assumes that a new direction has been found, which lies in extending working life and adopting a restricted understanding of active and productive ageing that has been reduced to work and work-like activities. Trying to make sense of this debate in terms of what it is trying to say about the purpose of a long life and how far it is an adaptation to a more balanced generational demographic can be difficult, confusing and subject to political interpretation. It focusses on continuity and immediacy, at the expense of distinctive lifecourse priorities. In terms of the alternative narratives available to us, it is perhaps the one that is least rooted in a stable basis on which to build a long life.

Work and ageing

The consensus that emerged in international social policy is of almost hegemonic proportions. It has become the common sense of national and international initiatives to claim that work is the obvious solution to population ageing (Moulaert & Biggs, 2013). Work, it is argued, sets up a virtuous economic circle in so far as rather than not paying so much tax and claiming social rights, such as a pension and health care, continuing to work longer would provide a larger tax base, boost the pool of productive workers and create fewer claims for social and health-care benefits. In the face of population ageing, working in later life has even be presented as an 'unavoidable obligation' (Reday-Mulvey, 2005: 195), a form of moral economy (Hendricks, 2005) for changed demographic conditions.

Two trends track these changes in the perceived relationship between work and adult ageing. The first concerns a shift from talking about active ageing to productive ageing. The second is a political economy critique of the disempowerment of older adults through forcible exclusion from working life.

Changing the narrative: from active to productive ageing

The concept of active ageing first came to prominence in contrast to ageing as disengagement (Havighurst, 1967; Cumming & Henry, 1961), both of which were interpretations of the same 'Kansas study' of 1960s Midwestern America. "Active ageing" is an approach that has its origins in the activity theory framework of that period, according to which 'psychological and social well-being could be enhanced by involvement in social roles and activities' (Estes, Biggs & Phillipson, 2003: 13). It received renewed attention in the late 1990s under the influence of the WHO, which was concerned with promoting a preventative, life-span approach to maintaining 'the highest possible quality of life for as long as possible, for the largest number of older people' (WHO, 1999). As originally envisaged, it encompassed a holistic approach that emphasised 'continuing participation in social, economic, cultural, spiritual and civic affairs not just the ability to be physically active or to participate in the labour force' (World Health Organization, 2002: 12). However, governments and policy makers have increasingly come to view 'active ageing' as a perspective that supports longer working lives and financial self-reliance in old age (Boudiny & Mortelmans, 2011; Moulaert & Biggs, 2013). This, suggest Boudiny and Mortelmans, 'comes as no surprise, given that the concept is rooted in the greying of the population and the related concerns about the sustainability of our social security systems' (2011: 8). Hence economic concerns have been placed at the core of active-ageing policies, with more holistic narratives being pushed to the margins. The interpretation of 'active ageing' promoted by the WHO has now largely been relegated to policy areas such as age-friendly urban planning and human and natural disasters. Much to the regret of early supporters (Walker, 2009; Walker & Maltby, 2012) holistic active ageing had elsewhere succumbed to its shrunken productivist cousin.

Following the Kansas study, the G8 Summit of 1997 (which was held just down the road in Denver) argued for a change in approach towards ageing: from a dependency-based to an active-labour market model (Walker, 1999). The summit's communique has formed a blueprint for subsequent policy development:

> We discussed the idea of 'active aging' – the desire and ability of many older people to continue work or other socially productive activities well into their later years, and agreed that old stereotypes of seniors as dependent should be abandoned. We considered new evidence suggesting that disability rates among seniors have declined in some countries while recognizing the wide variation in the health of older people. We discussed how our nations can

promote active aging of our older citizens with due regard to their individual choices and circumstances, including removing disincentives to labor force participation and lowering barriers to flexible and part-time employment that exist in some countries.

Communiqué, Summit of the Eight (G8, 1997)

Responding to the summit, the OECD produced a report in 1998 in which 'active ageing implies a high degree of flexibility in how individuals and families choose to spend their time over life in work, in learning, in leisure and in care-giving' (OECD, 1998: 14). OECD policy in the 1990s, then, marked a shift towards a more holistic vision of participation in society. Here, active ageing had two dimensions: to be able to lead a productive life and to be free to make personal choices in different arenas. However, following a review of pension policy in 21 member countries, the OECD position hardened to a more restricted and instrumental definition. The title of the synthesis report boils the argument down succinctly: *Ageing and employment policies: Live longer, work longer* (OECD, 2006), a position that has since been adopted in various degrees by both mature and emerging economies, being referred to as the productive-ageing approach.

This is not to say that the live longer, work longer approach is without its promoters, beyond what Vickerstaff (2010) has referred to as the discourse of labour economics. And here support originated from some unexpected sources. First reference to productive ageing occurred at the Salzberg conference of 1982 (Butler & Gleason, 1985) at which Betty Freiden, often cited as the founder of US feminism, opined that 'we can and must express and facilitate our personal and social productivity as we grow older', arising shortly afterwards from community work in Boston, Massachusetts. Here, *Bass, Caro and Chen (1993)* argued that in order to combat ageist stereotyping of older adults as a non-contributing drain on community resources, elders should be seen as productive members of society. Active and productive ageing was defined as 'any activity by an older individual that produces goods or services, or develops the capacity to produce them, whether they are to be paid for or not' (1993: 6). The reasoning behind this push was to make older adults more acceptable to the majority adult population by making them similar. In other words to 'make 'em like us' in both senses of that phrase – to be liked and to be the same. The notion of productive ageing was unashamedly economic in its foundation. Additional years of life had been viewed in terms of the increased opportunities for production, and it was predicted that 'rather than being seen as liabilities, older baby boomers will be deemed assets with an important role in sustaining economic growth' (Bass, 2000: 15). Bass and Caro (2001) also explicitly excluded activities that older adults might undertake for personal enrichment, such as meditation, religious reflection, and reminiscence, from their conception of being productive in later life. The purpose of a long life, then, is to be economically useful, or to support others in being so. And as such productive ageing provides ideological support to the neoliberal public policies outlined previously.

Empowerment and a new ageism

A second trend concerns the notion that rather than being a natural component of ageing, dependency was an enforced consequence of certain social conditions.

A key component to understanding the relationship between work and ageing is its malleability and historical contingency. In the course of the last century, retirement moved from being almost unknown to an increasingly early expectation, a 'third age' of active consumption, and then at its close, a source of concern. The UK experience serves as an example common to many developed economies. The idea of retiring at a fixed point in the lifecourse to enjoy the final years of life free from work and economic insecurity has been a relatively recent development (Phillipson, 2013). Historically speaking, the majority of workers experienced employment as 'a lifelong obligation that only sickness and infirmity could end' (Gilleard & Higgs, 2005: 5), with only elite public servants and those with private incomes having any prospect of a period of leisure as their lives drew to a close. With increased trade union and related Friendly Society activity during the later 19th century, limited mutual financial support became available for sickness and old age (Hardy, 2002). Even so, a comparatively high proportion of those who lived beyond the age of 65 remained in paid employment. For example, in 1891, 65% of British men over the age of 65 were in paid employment while, in 1931, the proportion was still as high as 48% (Thane, 2006). As the 20th century progressed, the proportion of the UK workforce covered by the new occupational pensions grew, from around one-third in 1956 to almost half the workforce by 1967 (Phillipson, 2013). In the context of changing social policy to accommodate a rising younger generation, the 1960s and '70s saw trends to encourage older workers to leave their jobs at earlier ages. Thus the current emphasis on longer working lives can be contrasted with policies towards older workers in previous decades when 'early retirement was being viewed as an entirely predictable and welcome development, a sign that the post-industrial society had now finally arrived' (Phillipson, 1998: 63–64).

The expectation that people should retire from employment at particular ages nevertheless had its own problems as it came under scrutiny from critical gerontologists of the period. Political economists of ageing had held concerns about the close link between retirement and poverty (Walker, 1980) and the role of retirement in fostering what Townsend (1981) termed the structured dependency of old age. Retirement, it was argued, fostered the 'popular perception of older people as being socially, politically and economically inactive' (Walker & Maltby, 2012: 118). Contrary to seeing pension eligibility as social achievement, it was presented as something that had largely been imposed on older adults by 'changes in the organization of work and in the kind of people wanted for work' (Townsend, 1981: 10). Viewed from this perspective, retirement or pension age eligibility was an arbitrary point for distinguishing the socially and economically useful from the dependent, thus stigmatising older people as passive recipients of welfare who were no longer capable of contributing to society (Walker, 1980). As with Freiden's (see Butler & Gleason, 1985) and Guillemard's (2007) feminist critiques, access to work was seen as the gateway to both meaningful social inclusion and workplace-based power relations. However, as the lengthening of retirement eligibility age and the work-based solution to all those extra years took shape, this traditional critical perspective has lost much of its force, leading to something of a crisis in the critical gerontological camp (van Dyk, 2014).

The approach to analysing the relationship between work and ageing adopted by these theorists marked a radical departure from preceding approaches in mainstream gerontology in that it focussed attention on how 'ageing' and 'retirement' were socially constructed phenomena, rather than biological facts of life. Therefore, they were contestable. However, as mainstream social policy began to catch up with many of the proposals made by critical gerontology – that age is not simply a matter of biological decline, there should be no compulsory retirement age and society should recognise age discrimination and elder abuse as explicit social problems, for example – it became clear that a new form of critique, paying greater attention to process rather than content was needed. The co-option and accompanying distortion of once radical concepts to justify the privatisation of social welfare and erosion of pension security, the requirement to work rather than the option of staying working and the increasing precarity that a new policy turn was bringing to ageing in mature economies made it a priority to re-evaluate what a contemporary critical approach might be. Little by little, it seemed that the aims of a radical gerontology had been turned inside out. They had become a means of legitimising the erosion of the conditions for a good life and were eclipsing what was both problematic about ageing and the special potential of a long life (Biggs, 2004; Calasanti, 2008; Holstein, 2011; Van Dyk, 2014). Combatting ageism, then, was not joined to a particular outcome – such as older workers being allowed to work for a longer part of their lives – but as an interaction between historical processes and changing power dynamics. These, it was argued, needed to take relations between age-generated lifecourse and externally imposed economic priorities into account. In many ways, it marks a shift from within-age thinking to between-age thinking.

Research accompanying the turn to work as a defining characteristic of social inclusion has focussed on whether there are differences between particular generations of workers and what older workers might actually want.

Are there generational differences in work attitudes?

Whether there are differences between older and younger workers is subject to opinion and mixed evidence. Studies arising from organisational behaviour have tended not to find marked age differences based on generational types, even though they at times uncritically adopt a named generation approach more often associated with marketing. By contrast gerontological studies have tended to be sceptical about the value of generational types, while finding age-based differences in attitudes to work. A critical review of generational differences in the workplace (Lyons & Kuron, 2014) indicates that studies are often simply descriptive and rarely reflect a theoretical understanding of the nature of age and generation. How-ever, they do conclude that when compared to previous generations, 'Evidence from time-lag and cross-sectional studies suggests that, despite a number of simi-larities, the generations in today's workplace differ in aspects of their personalities, work values and attitudes, leadership and teamwork preferences, leader behaviors, and career experiences' (2014: 149).

Lyons and Kuron argue for an overarching change in attitudes to work, reflect-ing a wider societal trend towards individualisation, which includes greater extroversion, personal conscientiousness and concern with self-esteem, but also greater neuroticism and narcissism. They point to an increased importance of material rewards and leisure, whereas a work ethic and the centrality of work in people's lives have been decreasing. 'Job satisfaction and organizational com-mitment appear lower among younger generations' (2014: 149) while IT skills, competitiveness and career mobility have increased as teamworking abilities have decreased. The results, they argue, support Twenge's (2006) depiction of an emer-gent "GenerationMe", who mark a continuing trend towards generations that are increasingly 'self-centered, agentic and high in self-esteem, but, paradoxically, suffer increased anxiety and depression' (Lyons & Kuron, 2014: 150). They con-clude that there is evidence that generational differences in the workplace are becoming more marked, but that it is difficult to demonstrate the degree to which they reflect personal observations of the behaviour of other generations or differ-ences in stereotypes.

Twenge et al. (2010) found generational differences in work values, with increasing leisure and extrinsic motivation and decreasing social and intrinsic reasons to value working life. They used a nationally representative sample of US high school seniors from 1976, 1991, and 2006, which they refer to as representing Baby Boomers, Generation X and Generation Me (also known as Generation Y, or Millennials). By collecting data across time, the researchers isolate generational differences from age differences, unlike cross-sectional studies, which cannot sep-arate the two. They found that whilst the value of leisure and out-of-work pursuits increased steadily over time, work centrality declined. Extrinsic motivators, such as status and money, peaked with Generation X but were still higher among Me generations than among boomers. They also noted that

> Contrary to popular press reports, GenMe does not favor altruistic work values (e.g., helping, societal worth) more than previous generations. Social values (e.g., making friends) and intrinsic values (e.g., an interesting, results-oriented job) were rated lower by GenMe than by Boomers.
>
> (2010: 152)

Cennamo and Gardner (2008) found that Baby Boomers reported better person-organisation value fit than Generation X and Generation Y, but there were no other generational differences. Both younger generations were more concerned with status and freedom at work, which the researchers put down to career stage differences rather than generational shifts per se. In a study by Fairlie (2013), North American baby boomers still in work reported slightly higher levels of meaningful work (self-actualising work, social impact, personal accomplishment) and work adjustment (job satisfaction, organisational commitment) than younger generations of workers.

Foster (2013) has identified different attitudes to work depending upon generation. Drawing on qualitative, narrative data from 52 interviews conducted between 2009 and 2011, she highlights the personal consequences of contemporary employment relations in Canada. These are characterised as including increasingly precarious work security, intensifying polarisation of wealth and shifting gender relations in families and in the workforce, plus the expansion of postsecondary education. She proposes that younger workers are more likely to construct and be associated with narratives of disaffection about work. In contrast, what the author terms ambivalent and faithful narratives were largely associated with older workers in later midlife. 'Narratives of disaffection tended to come from interviewees younger than 40, ambivalent narratives came *solely* from interviewees over age 45 and faithful narratives were most common among interviewees over 40 years of age' (2013: 7).

This is partly attributed to the different circumstances and work relations that, as generational groups, the workers experienced on entering working life and the changing nature of workplace relations. Younger workers showed a distanced relation to work, lack of identification with an employing organisation and an instrumental relation to working life, with 'life' and self-enhancement largely occurring elsewhere.

What Foster (2013) describes as an older worker's 'narrative of ambivalence', consisted of the worker seeing it as an essential moral and practical obligation but being unable 'to find the satisfaction, security, recognition and fulfilment others seemed to find in just doing it' (2013: 11). These workers found waning satisfaction with work but had difficulty imagining a life without it. They looked forward to retirement 'as a time to reclaim their lives' (Foster, 2013: 9). This was in stark contrast to those who could be described as having a 'faithful' work narrative 'where work time and personal time were almost indistinguishable' (8). Five basic themes connected faithful narratives to one another 'a reverence for work, respect for conventionally successful people, belief in the parity of work effort and reward, a strong connection drawn between personal and organizational goals and an emphasis on financial independence' (2013: 8).

Becton, Walker and Jones-Farmer (2014) explored actual workplace behaviour among baby boomers, generation X and millennials (N = 8,040, across two organisations). They found that differences were smaller than stereotypes might suggest but nevertheless there. Boomers were more likely to stay in the one job and were more job compliant than other groups, while Generation X was less likely to work overtime. Moore, Grunberg and Krause (2015) found that there were surprisingly few generational differences using college education as a proxy for social class. White-collar professionals and blue-collar production workers, working in the same company and from three different generational cohorts (Generation Y, Generation X and Baby Boomer) were compared. They found

> evidence for generational differences that confirms some of the common characterizations of Gen Y workers; however, this characterization was principally found within our professional subgroup of Gen Y employees . . . Gen Y employees . . . [were characterised] . . . as being less work-centric, more likely to value work and home, and more concerned with achieving work-life balance than 'Gen X' or 'Baby Boomer' employees.
>
> (2015: 357)

They suggest that other factors, such as workplace experiences and maturation, may shape current workplace expectations more than do generational differences, concluding that 'concern over generational differences may be limited to certain workplace expectations and to specific subgroups of employees' (2015: 346).

Are older workers better at certain things?

Studies of worker attitudes often leave the question open of whether certain groups of workers are better at some things than others. When it comes to age, there is some evidence that certain forms of ability, such as crystallised intelligence or accumulative knowledge actually appear to increase with age (Ackerman & Rolfhus, 1999). The experience of emotion also changes, with mature-age adults being more likely to let small problems go and being better at solving emotional conflicts (Charles & Carstensen, 2010). Skills that hinge on a greater understanding of systems and psychosocial aspects of working relationships may increase with age, highlighting the importance of an age-diverse workforce (Biggs & Lowenstein, 2011). To the age-specific skills of a mature workforce can be added greater reliability than younger workers. Older workers are less likely to engage in theft from their companies, be absent or quit their jobs (Broadbridge, 2001; Hedge, Borman & Lammlein, 2006). From a diversity perspective, it has been argued that older workers provide a depth of tacit knowledge both to fellow workers as well as clients and customers. A capacity to engage in problem solving and critical thinking at work with customers and co-workers also promotes innovation and supportive workplace practices in mature workers. In addition to this relational aspect to working, mature workers may have diverse social networks and social resources accumulated across their life spans, which organisations can leverage productively. The increased productivity of older workers has been most famously identified by BMW's experiment of employing older production line workers (Anderson, 2013). BMW made 70 small changes in the workplace to cut the chance of errors and reduce physical strain, such as special shoes, improved tools, new computer screens, wooden floors and rest and gym facilities. The project cost $50,000 and improved productivity by 7 percent, resulted in below average absenteeism, while the defect rate dropped to zero. In other words, 'It's no longer a project to aid the elderly; it's simply a fresh new plan to improve productivity' (Anderson, 2013: 488).

What do older workers want?

Whether older workers view the 'live-longer, work-longer' solution as an opportunity to 'age positively' or as a 'return to the bad old days where people "worked until they dropped"' (Davey & Davies, 2006: 23) remains a contested issue. Surveys of older workers' expectations provide some evidence that people are indeed considering working longer compared with previous generations of older workers. A report into Australian baby boomers' retirement expectations by AMP-NATCEM (2007) concluded that baby boomers are increasingly planning to stay at work or are looking for opportunities to re-enter the workforce. This echoed the results of a 2006 poll in which 40% of Australian boomer men and women surveyed said they expected to work past pension eligibility age (Hamilton & Hamilton, 2006). Surveys of older workers' retirement expectations, reporting in the decade up to 2013, covering Australia, the United Kingdom, and the United States, provide some evidence that people have been considering working longer (Hamilton & Hamilton, 2006; McNair, 2006; Walter, Jackson & Felmingham, 2008).

However, that people are considering working longer does not necessarily mean that they view this as a positive development and may reflect changing economic circumstances in which the task of ensuring adequate income in later life is now 'a far more complex process, with much more responsibility falling on the individual' (Hirsch, 2003: 7). Osberg (2005: 418) observes that changes in retirement expectations may simply 'be a consequence of the experience of greater economic insecurity during the working years', to which can be added an erosion of pension remuneration away from final salary and towards returns on contributions, and an extension of statutory retirement age (Vickerstaff & Cox, 2005). In the Australian context, workers in their 50s and early 60s have experienced greater economic insecurity, more unstable work histories and the hollowing out of full-time, continuous employment over the course of their working lives than preceding generations of older workers (Ozanne, 2009). Available research, from across the Anglosphere, suggests that financial need remains the key reason why many older adults expect to continue working, especially for those in lower-paid, lower-status occupations (Hamilton & Hamilton, 2006; Humphrey et al., 2003; Irving, Steels & Hall, 2005; Loretto & White, 2006; Quine, Bernard & Kendig, 2006).

Studies of retirement expectations since the global recession show that a large proportion of older workers are considering delaying their retirement because of the collapse in the value of their savings (Foot & Venne, 2011; Humpel et al., 2009; Pew Research Centre, 2010). Older people are more likely to report that they would quit working if they won the lottery (Highhouse, Zickar & Yankelevich, 2010), which may reflect a longstanding finding that routine or manual jobs, ones that involve being under a lot of stress or long hours, tend to become less tolerable as women and men grow older (McNair, 2006; Ginn & Arber, 2005; Smeaton, Vegeris & Sahin-Dikmen, 2009).

Those who remain in employment beyond typical UK retirement age tend to report higher levels of job satisfaction and more interesting work than other groups of workers (McNair, 2006; Smeaton et al., 2009). North American older workers who are still in employment report slightly higher levels of meaningful work and work adjustment than younger generations of workers (Fairlie, 2013). However, it has been argued that rather than showing that enjoyment of work increases with age, such findings may be evidence of "a strong survivor effect" (Vickerstaff, 2010: 873), whereby those most suited to contemporary work stay on, but others stop working, and 'a "shaking out" of the labour market in the midfifties, when many disaffected or demotivated people leave"' (McNair, 2006: 491).

At this point, important differences emerge between the dispositions of different groups of older workers towards longer working lives. In particular, Vickerstaff (2007) argues that 'there is a major distinction to be made between those who might want to continue working out of interest and those who feel that they must carry on working to sustain income' (2007: 593). This is reflected in Parry and Taylor's (2007) qualitative research into the attitudes of British older workers towards retirement. An important distinction emerges between what they call 'workers', on the one hand, and 'professionals and creatives', on the other. 'Workers' tend to regard paid employment primarily as a means to an end, necessary for supporting themselves and their families but not necessarily a source of satisfaction or personal fulfilment. These women and men mainly work in traditional working-class jobs and routine clerical roles. Paid work is clearly demarcated from their personal, family time and leisure, which is regarded as a separate sphere of life. Although this group holds a strong work ethic, they see retirement as a time when they can 'leave the employment treadmill, relax and enjoy life' (Parry & Taylor, 2007: 595). A separation of work and other parts of life is thus distinguished both in lifecourse time and in everyday time. Throughout their working lives few workers reported having much say over the type or hours of work they do and view 'getting the pension' as a form of reward and the beginning of a period of relative freedom in their use of time (see also, Loretto & Vickerstaff, 2013). As with Foster's (2013) 'ambivalent' baby boomers, Parry and Taylor's worker-respondents looked forward to postretirement as a time that reclaimed their lives from the drudgery of work. Professionals and creatives, on the other hand reflected a faith in work in which work and personal time became almost indistinguishable. The majority of this group reported finding the prospect of giving up paid work at retirement age illogical and sometimes even frightening. Their work is not just a job or a means to an end but an activity that was central to their personal identity and something they have no intention of stopping. These findings add detail to those of the 'Whitehall' longitudinal study of UK public servants (Stafford et al., 1998). Here workers lower in the hierarchy experienced stress, absenteeism and burnout that was associated with low levels of control over work processes and little room for autonomous decision making. Higher-level public servants also reported stress, but this was more likely to be interpreted positively in the context of personal autonomy and discretion on work-related activities.

Australian research (McGann et al., 2015) indicated that older workers expressed at least four different orientations towards continued working. Some were 'jaded by work,' feeling betrayed by changes in the job market. Others saw a changed work-life balance as conducive to self-development. A third group could not imagine life at any age without work, while a fourth group had no choice but to work. A combination of workplace ageism and a progressive credentialism and casualisation of work opportunities were associated with negative reactions to work in later life.

When it comes to discovering what older workers want, the answer seems to lie in a combination of changing workplace conditions, and social class position as well as in generational difference. Rather than looking at worker characteristics, a more fruitful question might be to critically examine how work can be adapted to the needs of older and other workers. Vickerstaff (2010: 873) describes 'a conundrum in existing research on what older workers want' in that many workers express a willingness to consider working longer but want to change the terms under which they work. Their willingness to continue working depends upon the terms being right and, in particular, on being able to have greater work-life balance or change to more interesting jobs. How women and men describe the factors that will influence their willingness to work reveals a changing orientation towards it among those in a position to choose whether or not to continue working. Although a significant proportion of older workers are prepared to consider working past retirement age, few are willing to continue working in the same jobs or to the same extent as earlier in their working lives (Vickerstaff, 2010). For British workers, issues of job satisfaction, job quality and work-life balance take on increasing importance as the possibility of work ending comes into view (Smeaton et al., 2009). Cennamo and Gardner (2008) observed that US workers with a lack of fit between personal and organisational values reported reduced job satisfaction and commitment and an increased intention to leave across three generational groups. The values held by individuals were, however, less important for outcomes than perceptions of what organisations offered their workers. In Finland, research by Manninen (2011) has shown that even if workers have positive abilities and motivation towards work, a poorly adapted workplace culture will discourage recruitment and retention of mature workers. Those with a positive disposition to continuing working often want to reduce their working hours or change the type of work that they do as a condition of extending their working lives (Irving et al., 2005; McNair, 2006; Vickerstaff, 2010). This may mean being able to downshift to a job with reduced hours and responsibilities (Irving et al., 2005; Loretto & White, 2006) or being able to take up a second career in a new line of work they find constructive and enjoyable. In particular, older workers report a strong preference for working on a part-time or flexible basis and 'actively seek a balance between work and other aspects of their lives including family care, voluntary work and educational pursuits' (Gardiner et al., 2007: 477). As Vickerstaff (2010) found in her study of the attitudes of older workers in Scotland to the prospect of working past retirement age, those who were prepared to continue working felt that 'at this time in their lives employment would take a back seat and would need to fit around other aspects of life and not *vice versa* as had been the case for much of their working years' (2010: 874).

It is important here not to lose sight of the experience of mature age itself as a factor influencing decisions on whether to work. Fasbender et al.'s (2014) study of postretirement working indicated that there is a close relationship between the likelihood of working and the psychological experience of ageing. Using longitudinal data from the German Ageing Survey, they found that both positive and negative dimensions predicted whether retirees approached or avoided a return to work. Retirees who experienced ageing either as social loss or as a time of personal skill development were more likely to engage in postretirement employment a decade later. However, those who experienced ageing as gaining self-knowledge were less likely to engage in postretirement employment. Aquino et al. (1996) had suggested that employment can provide social support for older people, although whether this is because work has had a negative effect on other forms of support is unclear. In Fasbender et al.'s (2014) study, older adults who had experienced a loss of social contact and stimulation were more likely to seek social support at work and were likely to engage in employment to compensate for their experienced losses and feelings of being less needed. For those who experienced later life as a time of personal growth, further employment acted as a vehicle by which to further expand their professional knowledge and skills. Personal growth in the sense of developing knowledge and skill is contrasted with self-knowledge, however. For those in this last group, self-knowledge, characterised as 'fully realizing the benefits of their ageing process', was best achieved by alternatives to work, which was itself seen as preventing self-discovery and was therefore avoided. McGann et al.'s (2015) respondents who wanted to return to work, also expressed concerns about the low level, poor quality and unpredictability of employment they were offered in later midlife.

Taken together, these studies indicate that age priorities, though differing between groups of mature age workers, influence not only a qualified willingness to work but also changes in the forms of work deemed desirable.

The fetishisation of work

Work, then, has become a marker of a specific form of economic continuity with little room for positive discontinuity. It has increasingly come to be seen as a container for activity, most notably productive capacity, and as a means of social inclusion. The medium through which this has taken place has been predominantly social policy. It's dynamic, a form of denial through a guiding myth of agelessness, makes lifecourse and intergenerational distinctiveness hard to include within its narrative structure, rendering them difficult to negotiate.

Unfortunately, the productivist solution to the question of a long life ultimately represents a capitulation to the values that have contributed to the negative social construction of ageing in the first place (Estes et al., 2003). In other words, a person's social value rests on a restricted ability to engage in work or activities that mimic working life. Social value is returned to the older adult only insofar as he or she is not dependent, thereby reinforcing instrumental ideologies that may fail to accommodate changing lifecourse priorities. The policy consensus around work marks a shift away from a holistic approach to the inclusion of older adults to one which focusses almost entirely on employment as the road to social inclusion for older adults. Work, from the perspective of purpose and intergenerational relations, appears as a borrowed and doubly inauthentic solution to the question of what to do with a long life – first, as an extension of what had come to be seen as a different lifecourse-specific episode, and second, as importing politics that views ageing as an economic problem that arose from elsewhere and is used to mask other forms of social inequality.

Work, then, as the solution to the question of a long life has several disadvantages. First, it is unclear how far it fits with specific lifecourse tasks or whether it is simply 'more of the same' importing age and instrumental priorities from elsewhere. It therefore represents a form of present rather than lifetime centredness. Second, work is assumed to be a relatively age-neutral environment – that it is one's ability to compete, regardless of social and age categories, on the same ground of productivity that determines social value. Third, it is very much a 'within later life' position in the sense that it may form a policy answer to 'what to do with older people' but doesn't readily place the extension of working life within the context of wider intergenerational processes and social inequalities. Finally, and perhaps most tellingly, work can be used as a means of avoiding the challenge of a long life, of confrontation with one's intrinsic rather than extrinsic value, when other props to identity are stripped away. It does not allow for positive discontinuities, except in productive differences identified between generational groups. Even here, it is unclear whether positive othering occurs, as all working groups are judged by the same yardstick, ultimately suggesting generational competition. Work, then, does not emerge as an adaptation to a longer life at all; rather it is simply a continuation of existing strategies. It is more of the same.

References

Ackerman, P. L., & Rolfhus, E. L. (1999). The locus of adult intelligence: Knowledge, abilities, and non-ability traits. *Psychology and Aging*, *14*, 314–330.

AMP-NATCEM. (2007). *Baby boomers–doing it for themselves*. Income and Wealth Report Issue 16. Canberra, Australia: University of Canberra.

Anderson, L. B. (2013). How frames present BMW as embracing an aging workforce. *Public Relations Review*, *39*(5), 484–490.

Aquino, J. A., Russell, D. W., Cutrona, C. E., & Altmaier, E. M. (1996). Employment status, social support, and life satisfaction among the elderly. *Journal of Counseling Psychology*, *43*(4), 480–489.

Bass, S. A. (2000). Emergence of the third age: Toward a productive aging society. *Journal of Aging & Social Policy*, *11*(2–3), 7–17.

Bass, S. A., & Caro, F. G. (2001). Productive aging: A conceptual framework. In N. Morrow-Howell, J. Hinterlong & M. Sherraden (Eds.), *Productive aging: Concepts and challenges* (pp. 37–78). Baltimore, MD: Johns Hopkins University Press.

Bass, S. A., Caro, F. J., & Chen, Y. P. (1993). *Achieving a productive aging society*. Westport, CT: Auburn House.

Becton, J., Walker, J., & Jones-Farmer, A. (2014). Generational differences in workplace behaviour. *Journal of Applied Social Psychology*, *44*(3), 175–189.

Biggs, S. (2004). Age, gender, narratives, and masquerades. *Journal of Aging Studies*, *18*(1), 45–58.

Biggs, S., Carstensen, L., & Hogan, P. (2012). Social capital, lifelong learning and social innovation. In J. Beard, S. Biggs, D. Bloom, L. Fried, P. Hogan, A. Kalache & J. Olshansky (Eds.), *Global population ageing: Peril or promise?* (Working Paper No.89, pp. 39–41). Geneva, Switzerland: World Economic Forum.

Biggs, S., & Lowenstein, A. (2011). *Generational intelligence: A critical approach to age relations.* New York, NY: Routledge.

Boudiny, K., & Mortelmans, D. (2011). A critical perspective: Towards a broader understanding of "active ageing". *Sensoria: A Journal of Mind, Brain & Culture, 7*(1), 8–14.

Broadbridge, A. (2001). Ageism in retailing: Myth or reality? In I. Golver & M. Branine (Eds.), *Ageism in work and employment* (pp. 153–174). Burlington, VT: Ashgate.

Butler, R. N., & Gleason, H. P. (1985). *Productive aging.* New York, NY: Springer Publishing Company.

Calasanti, T. (2008). A feminist confronts ageism. *Journal of Aging Studies, 22*(2), 152–157.

Cennamo, L., & Gardner, D. (2008). Generational differences in work values, outcomes and person-organisation values fit. *Journal of Managerial Psychology, 23*, 891–906.

Charles, S. T., & Carstensen, L. L. (2010). Social and emotional aging. *Annual Review of Psychology, 61*, 383–409.

Commonwealth of Australia. (2015). The intergenerational report. Retrieved from www.treasury.gov.au/PublicationsAndMedia/Publications/2015/2015-Intergenerational-Report

Cumming, E., & Henry, W. E. (1961). *Growing old, the process of disengagement.* New York, NY: Basic Books.

Davey, J., & Davies, M. (2006). Work in later life-opportunity or threat? *Social Policy Journal of New Zealand, 27*, 20–37.

Estes, C. L., Biggs, S., & Phillipson, C. (2003). *Social theory, social policy, and ageing: A critical introduction.* Berkshire: Open University Press.

European Union. (2012). European year of active ageing & intergenerational solidarity 2012. Retrieved May 8, 2017, http://www.age-platform.eu/images/stories/EY2012_Campaign.pdf

Fairlie, P. (2013). Age and generational differences in work psychology: Facts, fictions, and meaningful work. In J. Field, R. J. Burke & C. L. Cooper (Eds.), *The Sage handbook of aging, work and society* (pp. 186–208). London, England: Sage.

Fasbender, U., Deller, J., Wang, M., & Wiernik, B. M. (2014). Deciding whether to work after retirement: The role of the psychological experience of aging. *Journal of Vocational Behavior, 84*(3), 215–224.

Foot, D., & Venne, R. (2011). The long goodbye: Age, demographics, and flexibility in retirement. *Canadian Studies in Population, 38*(3–4), 59–74.

Foster, K. R. (2013). Disaffection rising? Generations and the personal consequences of paid work in contemporary Canada. *Current Sociology, 61*(7), 931–948.

G8. (1997). Communiqué from the Denver summit of the eight, Denver, USA, June 20–22. Retrieved May 8, 2017, from www.g8.utoronto.ca/summit/1997denver/g8final.htm

Gardiner, J., Stuart, M., Forde, C., Greenwood, I., MacKenzie, R., & Perrett, R. (2007). Work–life balance and older workers: Employees' perspectives on retirement transitions following redundancy. *The International Journal of Human Resource Management, 18*(3), 476–489.

Gilleard, C., & Higgs, P. (2005). *Contexts of ageing: Class, cohort and community.* Cambridge, UK: Polity Press.

Ginn, J., & Arber, S. (2005). Longer working: Imposition or opportunity? Midlife attitudes to work across the 1990s. *Quality in Ageing and Older Adults, 6*(2), 26–35.

Guillemard, A. M. (2007). The advent of a flexible life-course and the reconfiguration of welfare. In J. Goul Andersen, A. M. Guillemard, P. H. Jensen & B. Pfau-Effinger (Eds.), *Changing face of welfare* (pp. 131–146). England: University of Bristol, Policy Press.

Hamilton, S. F., & Hamilton, M. A. (2006). School, work, and emerging adulthood. In M. A. Arnett, J. Jensen & J. F. Tanner (Eds.), *Emerging adults in America: Coming of age in the 21st century* (pp. 257–277). Washington, DC: American Psychological Association.

Hardy, M. A. (2002). The transformation of retirement in twentieth-century America: From discontent to satisfaction. *Generations, 26*(2), 9–16.

Havighurst, R. (1967). *A crossnational study of life styles and patterns of aging.* Proceedings of the Annual Meeting of the Gerontological Society, 43. American Psychological Association, Washington, DC.

Hedge, J. W., Borman, W. C., & Lammlein, S. E. (2006). *The aging workforce: Realities, myths, and implications for organizations.* Washington, DC: American Psychological Association.

Hendricks, J. (2005). Moral economy and ageing. In M. L. Johnson (Ed.), *The Cambridge handbook of age and ageing* (pp. 510–517). Cambridge, England: Cambridge University Press.

Highhouse, S., Zickar, M. J., & Yankelevich, M. (2010). Would you work if you won the lottery? Tracking changes in the American work ethic. *Journal of Applied Psychology, 95*(2), 349–357.

Hirsch, D. (2003). *Crossroads after 50: Improving choices in work and retirement.* Bristol, England: Policy Press.

Holstein, M. (2011). Cultural ideals, ethics, and agelessness: A critical perspective on the third age. In D. C. Carr & K. Komp (Eds.), *Gerontology in the era of the third age* (pp. 225–242). New York, NY: Springer Publishing Company.

Humpel, N., O'Loughlin, K., Wells, Y., & Kendig, H. (2009). Ageing of baby boomers in Australia: Evidence informing actions for better retirement. *Australian Journal of Social Issues, 44*(4), 399–415.

Humphrey, A., Costigan, P., Pickering, K., Stratford, N., & Barnes, M. (2003). *Factors affecting the labour market participation of older workers* (No. 200). Leeds, England: Department for Work and Pensions.

Irving, P., Steels, J., & Hall, N. (2005). *Factors affecting the labour market participation of older workers: Qualitative research* (Vol. 281). Leeds, England: Department for Work and Pensions.

Loretto, W., & Vickerstaff, S. (2013). The domestic and gendered context for retirement. *Human Relations, 66*(1), 65–86.

Loretto, W., & White, P. (2006). Work, more work and retirement: Older workers' perspectives. *Social Policy and Society, 5*(4), 495–506.

Lyons, S., & Kuron, L. (2014). Generational differences in the workplace: A review of the evidence and directions for future research. *Journal of Organizational Behavior, 35*(S1), S139–S157.

Manninen, O. (2011). Willingness and ability to keep on working: Care work and care working communities compared with 10,000 other tasks and working communities. In O. Manninen (Ed.), *The 13th international conference on combined actions and combined effects of environmental factors.* Paper presented at Work among the elderly: Tampere, Finland, September (pp. 9–31). Tampere, Finland: Printing Company.

McGann, M., Bowman, D., & Kimberley, H., & Biggs, S. (2015). *Too old to work, too young to retire*. Research Insight Report. Melbourne: Brotherhood of St Laurence.

McNair, S. (2006). How different is the older labour market? Attitudes to work and retirement among older people in Britain. *Social Policy and Society*, *5*(4), 485–494.

Moore, S., Grunberg, L., & Krause, A. J. (2015). Generational differences in workplace expectations: A comparison of production and professional workers. *Current Psychology*, *34*(2), 346–362.

Moulaert, T., & Biggs, S. (2013). International and European policy on work and retirement: Reinventing critical perspectives on active ageing and mature subjectivity. *Human Relations*, *66*(1), 23–43.

OECD. (1988). *Ageing populations: The social policy implications*. Paris, France: OECD.

OECD. (1998). *Maintaining prosperity in an ageing society: The OECD study on the policy implications of ageing*. France: Organisation for Economic Cooperation and Development.

OECD. (2006). *Ageing and employment policies: Live longer, work longer*. Paris, France: Author.

Osberg, L. (2005). Work and well-being in an aging society. *Canadian Public Policy/Analyse de Politiques*, *31*(4), 413–420.

Ozanne, E. (2009). Negotiating identity in late life: Diversity among Australian baby boomers. *Australian Social Work*, *62*(2), 132–154.

Parry, J., & Taylor, R. F. (2007). Orientation, opportunity and autonomy: Why people work after state pension age in three areas of England. *Ageing and Society*, *27*(4), 579–598.

Pew Research Center. (2010). Baby boomers approach 65: Glumly. Retrieved September 25, 2015, from www.pewsocialtrends.org/2010/12/20/baby-boomers-approach-65-glumly/

Phillipson, C. (1998). *Reconstructing old age: New agendas in social theory and practice*. London, England: Sage.

Phillipson, C. (2013). *Ageing*. Cambridge and Malden, MA: Polity Press.

Quine, S., Bernard, D., & Kendig, H. (2006). Understanding baby boomer's expectations and plans for their retirement: Findings from a qualitative study. *Australasian Journal on Ageing*, *25*(3), 145–150.

Reday-Mulvey, G. (2005). *Working beyond 60: Key policies and practices in Europe*. New York, NY: Springer Publishing Company.

Smeaton, D., Vegeris, S., & Sahin-Dikmen, M. (2009). *Older workers: Employment preferences, barriers and solutions*. Manchester, England: Equality and Human Rights Commission.

Stafford, M., Hemingway, H., Stansfeld, S. A., Brunner, E., & Marmot, M. (1998). Behavioural and biological correlates of physical functioning in middle aged office workers: The UK Whitehall II study. *Journal of Epidemiology and Community Health*, *52*(6), 353–358.

Thane, P. (2006). Women and ageing in the twentieth century. *L'Homme: Zeitschrift für Feministische Geschichtswissenschaft*, *17*(1), 59–74.

Townsend, P. (1981). The structured dependency of the elderly: A creation of social policy in the twentieth century. *Ageing and Society*, *1*(1), 5–28.

Twenge, J. M. (2006). *Generation me: Why today's young Americans are more confident, assertive, entitled – and more miserable than ever before*. New York, NY: Free Press.

Twenge, J. M., Campbell, S. M., Hoffman, B. J., & Lance, C. E. (2010). Generational differences in work values: Leisure and extrinsic values increasing, social and intrinsic values decreasing. *Journal of Management*, *36*(5), 1117–1142.

UK Government Department of Work and Pensions. (2017). Fuller working lives. Retrieved May 12, 2017 https://www.gov.uk/government/publications/fuller-working-lives-a-partnership-approach.

US Department of Health and Human Services. (1997). Active aging: a shift in the paradigm. Retrieved July 16, 2015 http://aspe.hhs.gov/daltcp/reports/actaging.pdf

van Dyk, S. (2014). The appraisal of difference: Critical gerontology and the active ageing paradigm. *Journal of Aging Studies, 31,* 93–103.

Vickerstaff, S. (2007). What do older workers want? Gradual retirement. *Social and Public Policy Review, 1*(1), 1–13.

Vickerstaff, S. (2010). Older workers: The "unavoidable obligation" of extending our working lives? *Sociology Compass, 4*(10), 869–879.

Vickerstaff, S., & Cox, J. (2005). Retirement and risk: The individualisation of retirement experiences? *The Sociological Review, 53*(1), 77–95.

Walker, A. (1980). The social creation of poverty and dependency in old age. *Journal of Social Policy, 9*(1), 49–75.

Walker, A. (1999). *Managing an ageing workforce: A guide to good practice.* Dublin, Ireland: European Foundation for the Improvement of Living and Working Conditions.

Walker, A. (2009). Commentary: The emergence and application of active aging in Europe. *Journal of Aging & Social Policy, 21,* 75–93.

Walker, A., & Maltby, T. (2012). Active ageing: A strategic policy solution to demographic ageing in the European Union. *International Journal of Social Welfare, 21*(1), S117–S130.

Walter, M., Jackson, N., & Felmingham, B. (2008). Keeping Australia's older workers in the labour force: A policy perspective. *Australian Journal of Social Issues, 43*(2), 291–309.

World Bank. (1994). *Averting the old-age crisis: Policies to protect the old and promote growth.* New York, NY: Oxford University Press.

World Health Organization. (1999). *Ageing: Exploding the myths.* Geneva, Switzerland: Author.

World Health Organization. (2002). *Active ageing: A policy framework.* Second World Assembly on Aging. Madrid, Spain: World Health Organization.

4   Is work good or bad for health?

Key themes

- Policy narratives have associated work with continued good health
- Evidence suggests both work and retirement can be good for health
- The quality of transition from work to non-work has implications for well-being
- While good health can lead to continued working, work does not in itself create good health
- The changing nature of work has created new threats to well-being
- Both daily life and the lifetime have become commodified, affecting work-life balance

Policy, health and older working

In 1998, the OECD, cognisant of projected increases in pensions and health expenditure, made the following statement. Working longer, it was argued, was connected to health, since 'those who work longer enjoy better health in their old age' (OECD, 1998: 14–15). In 1999, the European Commission also claimed that extending working life 'is one important way of adding life to longer years' (Commission of the European Communities, 1999: 21). During the same period, advocates of productive ageing emphasised how, with gains in health and longevity, 'people now have the potential for remaining productive later in life than in the past' (Bass, Caro & Chen, 1993: 250). Tapping into the productive potential of older people, they argued, would not only bring economic benefits for society but would also enhance quality of life in old age since health and productivity 'go hand and hand and deteriorate together' (Butler & Gleason, 1985: xii). A new literature emerged documenting 'the multiple ways people contribute to their own health, to their families and communities, and to society as they age' (Johnson & Mutchler, 2014: 95).

These two discourses, arising from the political and the gerontological, make a clear link between work, ageing and health. They appear to make a causal connection, in so far as working life is assumed to be directly responsible for health in later life and that this relationship is a positive one. However, in the 1990s, evidence on this relationship was slim, and the dominant trend, at least in the developed economies, was for older workers to retire before the statutory pension age (Phillipson, 1998). Research on health and ageing largely concentrated on maintenance and quality of life after retirement (Victor, 1991; Rowe & Kahn, 1997), partly because state pension eligibility was then the principal marker of the transition into older age. Academic work on the relationship between health and employment had been almost universal in reporting the negative effects of work, as a principal site of exploitation (Beynon, 1984) and as a contributory factor in health inequality (Marmot et al., 1997). By the early 1990s, with the growing dominance of neoliberal economics, the sociology of work had fallen into what contemporaries thought of as a terminal decline (Phillipson, personal communication). While there was some psychological evidence that working life could benefit well-being through social contact and structuring everyday experience (Warr & Wall, 1975; Warr, 1997), this largely impacted because it was perceived to be counterintuitive. Work, it seemed, had some benefits after all over and above income, though these were secondary. Warr's work used these additional factors as a variable allowing him to discriminate between forms of work that increased or decreased social happiness, rather than claiming a unidirectional relationship between work, positive social and health effects and overall happiness itself (Warr, 2007) – in other words, demonstrating that degrees of social participation and well-being can be used to measure good working environments rather than work itself creating them.

The proposed causal association between work and good health, however, continues to be used to support arguments for longer working and reduced eligibility for pensions and, as such, has become a debate that is deeply ideological. This position is proposed by the Centre for Market Reform of Education and the Institute of Economic Affairs (Sahlgren, 2013), for example, while an association between poor health and work stokes alternative political positions, such as that of the UK Trades Union Congress (2012).

Nevertheless, an association between well-being and work, or work-like activities, has been maintained in international policy discourse, particularly in European policy. In 2012, for example, the introduction to the European Year of Active Ageing and Solidarity Between Generations stated that empowering older people to age in good health and to contribute more actively to the labour market and their communities would be a core element in reducing public expenditure (European Union, 2012). The concern here is twofold. First, if older people stay healthy, they will contribute to the economy and not draw down on health and social benefits. Second, echoing *Bass et al.'s (1993)* US work on productive ageing in community settings, productive ageing reduces the threat of population ageing to younger generations. The twinning of solidarity and ageing, characteristic of EU social policy, reflects a continuing fear that the social contract between generations that supports the payment of pensions and health care for the old may break down.

The association between health, ageing and social inclusion through work has been taken further by the advocates of a longevity dividend. Rather than creating a drain on economic growth or longevity deficit, a healthy, long life, it is argued, can actually present an opportunity for continuing prosperity (Olshansky et al., 2006; Butler et al., 2008; Miller, 2009; Olshansky, Beard & Börsch-Supan, 2012). Here, it is claimed that the extension of healthy life creates wealth for individuals and the nations in which they live. As Olshansky et al. (2006) state,

> If we succeed in slowing ageing by seven years, the age-specific risk of death, frailty, and disability will be reduced by approximately half at every age . . . creating . . . Social, economic, and health bonuses for both individuals and entire populations – a dividend that would begin with generations currently alive and continue.
>
> (2006: 35)

While in a less ambitious form, the European Innovation Partnership on Active and Healthy Ageing (EIP-AHA, 2012), an initiative to combine research and business interests, took this idea up at the level of policy and development.

> The partnership brings together public and private stakeholders across boards and sectors to accelerate the uptake of innovation, with the goal of increasing by two years the average healthy life years (HLY) of EU citizens by 2020. The EIP-AHA pursues a 'triple win' for the EU: by improving health status and quality of life of older people; by improving efficiency and sustainability of health systems; and by fostering the competitiveness of EU industry working in innovative age and health related products and services.
>
> (EIP-AHA, 2012: 3)

So while the original policy position maintained that work leads to health in later life, the practical outcome has been to associate health with the ability to continue working. The policy and ideological consequences in this relatively small semantic shift are, however, significant. The first would privilege labour economics and the mechanisms that incentivise staying in work. The second would draw attention to ways in which people throughout the lifecourse can be encouraged to stay healthy, so that they can then maintain longer and more productive lives. One sees a long life as problematic unless costs can be reduced, the other as a potential benefit to economic growth.

The relationship between work, health and later life

So what is the evidence of an association between work, health and later life? The intervening years, since the original OECD statement, have seen a renewed interest in research in ageing and work (Field, Burke & Cooper, 2013). Could it be that working life had become more advantageous to health? Or that the relationship between work and well-being had experienced a radical flip between traditional working age and work in late life – with a negative being turned into a positive experience for older workers?

In 2002, a working group from the Australian Psychological Society reviewed the existing evidence on the relationship between physical and mental health, work and unemployment. They concluded that

> Employed people enjoy better mental health than do most unemployed people and longitudinal research findings support the conclusion that this is because employment status affects mental health. However, whether the experience of work is beneficial or detrimental depends on the quality of the work experience. The claim that even bad jobs are better for psychological wellbeing than unemployment is not supported by research.
>
> (Winefield, 2000: 2)

The working group pointed out that status and social inclusion in western societies depends on a reliable and secure work income, which then allows access to desired activities and goods, plus culture-bound social value as a successful member of society. This sets up an additional tension where unpaid work at home and remuneration for paid employment are heavily gendered. They observed that increases in the prevalence of casual, contract labour had had adverse effects on family life, the experience of work and future career paths. Downsizing, the stripping out of middle-layer workers and increasing workloads had adverse effects on health, psychological well-being and productivity. Job loss in middle age, the working group maintained, had been shown to be the most damaging, more so than unemployment for the young.

Research by the UK-based Work Foundation (Brinkley et al., 2010) on the changing nature of working life, indicated that early hopes of a 'knowledge economy' providing a less stressful workplace with greater autonomy and a better work-life balance had not been fulfilled in practice. They concluded that

> While the physical nature of work has changed many argue that increased work intensity, increased discretion and intellectual demands imposed on workers in the knowledge economy are key contributing factors to the cause and nature of work-related ill health. Indeed, the prevalence of work-related stress has increased alongside the numbers of knowledge workers.
>
> (2010: 14)

The Work Foundation further maintained that employment trends had moved towards greater polarisation. There were more high-skill, high-remuneration and low-skill, low-remuneration jobs, with a stripping out of middle-range employment. As such, these findings conformed to the scenario modelling of the UK Commission of Employment and Skills (2014) for workplace needs in 2030. The commission outlined four scenarios, including forced flexibility, skills activism, the great divide (in forms of inequality) and innovation adaptation. Each of these scenarios had predicted increased polarisation in terms of skill and remuneration, with reduced social benefits as a result of zero-hour contracting and the erosion of middle-level work due principally to the automation of white-collar work. In addition, Vaughan-Jones and Barham (2009) have argued that on current projections, the future health of the workforce to 2030 included a more obese population, living with more long-term conditions (such as chronic heart disease, mental illness, musculoskeletal disorders, diabetes and asthma) and that workers would have more caring responsibilities for others.

When it comes to older workers, Holstein (2011) reminds us that while 'The message is that we are only as old as we feel, that 60 is the new 40', for many people, the reality of spending more years of their life in the workforce may be far removed from the agentic positive experience envisaged by discourses of active and productive ageing. Indeed older workers appear trapped between a stripping out of many existing jobs and falling pension incomes. With rising pension ages and the collapse in the value of retirement savings in defined contribution plans since the global financial crisis (Ekerdt, 2010: 75), many people may have little choice over whether, and how, they continue working. As Calasanti and King (2011: 75) highlight, the global economic recession has 'made the Third Age descriptor even less likely for future retirees'. The economic downturn in the United States left more than twice as many Americans aged 55 and older unemployed in July 2009 compared with November 2007, while the number of age-discrimination claims jumped by more than 25% during the first year of the recession (Calasanti & King, 2011: 76). Taylor (2010) points to rising underemployment among workers over 50 in Europe as further evidence of the 'significant constraints on the choices of older workers' (2010: 547). This is supported by studies of the employment options available to older workers in the UK that suggest the option of reconfiguring work in ways that better meet their preferences is still distant for most older workers (Loretto, Lain & Vickerstaff, 2013). McGann et al.'s (2015) Australian study reports both a difficulty in finding appropriate work among people who find themselves 'underemployed' and reports of increasing age discrimination in both workplaces and job-finding agencies. Lain's (2012) analysis of working past 65 in the UK suggests that the pervasiveness of ageism in the labour market is restricting job opportunities in later life to lower-status sales, service and elementary occupations with very low weekly wages and often unsociable hours of employment. As Phillipson (2013) warns, the danger is that 'people will be increasingly caught between insecure work on the one side and an increasingly insecure retirement on the other' (2013: 77). These findings would suggest that contemporary working life is becoming more stressful as the forms and quality of work change, with a particular anxiety connected to attitudes towards older workers.

In their survey of "Quality of Work, Wellbeing and Retirement", Siegrist and Wahrendorf (2013) offer a cautionary analysis of the health benefits of longer working lives under conditions of degraded working environments. They point to several examples of how continued working in physically or psychosocially stressful jobs can increase the risk of musculoskeletal disorders and cardiovascular disease in later life. For example, working in physically stressful jobs involving restricted posture, heavy lifting or repetitive movements can increase the risk of premature retirement due to disability by 50 to 100%. It is estimated that close to half of all workers in Europe are exposed to these conditions, although the risk of exposure is particularly high among lower-status and lower-skilled workers in the construction, agriculture, transport and mining sectors. Psychosocial stressors included having low control over work in the face of high demands, being treated unfairly by mangers or colleagues, and lack of reciprocity. These are health risks encountered daily by many workers. Jobs characterised by these sources of psychosocial stress are associated with elevated risks of depression, diabetes, and several other forms of cardiovascular disease, leading Siegrist and Wahrendorf (2013) to conclude that 'retirement is experienced as a relief from the burden of work by a significant proportion of the workforce' (2013: 320).

It appears from the above that working life had not improved between the 1990s and the 20 teens, and if anything, the negative associations with health have been growing. It is important in this context to note that the key policy comparison for older workers extends to the effects of working life and of retirement and not the more general context of unemployment. It is to the role of retirement on health that we now turn in more detail.

Work, retirement and health

The Australian Psychological Society's report (2002) concludes that retirement can be beneficial or deleterious depending on several factors, particularly, health, financial security and an individual's perceived control over the decision. Indeed, older workers may be subject to a contradictory set of expectations, with government encouragement for delayed retirement standing alongside community pressure to leave work to make room for younger workers.

Data from the European Study of Health Ageing and Retirement in Europe (SHARE), covering upwards of 35,000 people aged 50 years and over in 15 EU countries, showed a strong correlation between quality of work and intended retirement from work, with poor working environments occasioning earlier exit from the workforce (Siegrist & Wahrendorf, 2009). While Tuomi et al. (2001) and Westerlund et al. (2009) reported that poor quality of work both reduces the health and well-being of employees and increases the likelihood of retirement. Westerlund et al. (2010) have also shown that, among French workers in the energy supply industry, retirement is associated with a lessening of fatigue and small decreases in depression. There are also gender differences between older workers and their intention to retire early. Negative perceptions of work and low life satisfaction were associated with early retirement intentions among women, whereas men cited poor self-rated work ability and perceived poor health as reasons for leaving work (Von Bonsdorff et al., 2009). Wahrendorf et al. (2015) have also found that willingness to volunteer in retirement is related to the quality of working life in the middle years.

A study of cognitive functioning (cited by Field et al., 2013), covering 13 countries, indicates that 'work provided an environment that kept individuals functioning optimally' when compared to retirement: 'Working maintains one's social and personality skills, the routine of getting up in the morning, dealing with other people, and being prompt, dependable and trustworthy' (2013: 10). Work, in other words, provides the psychosocial discipline necessary to continue working. Wickrama et al. (2013) used a subsample of 8,524 older adults who participated in the US Health and Retirement Study from 1998 to 2008 and were 62 years or older in 1998. After controlling for age and background characteristics, they concluded that work status and health outcomes interacted with each other in terms of immediate memory over time, physical disability and depressive symptoms. They point out that in previous research 'Mixed findings about the directional association between working status and health outcomes in later years may be attributed to several methodological reasons' (2013: 811). They conclude that memory loss is more closely connected to differential processes of ageing than level of working, but that physical disability and mental health problems created a reciprocal association, in a cycle whereby poor health prompts reduced work, which then exacerbates continued negative health status, claiming that 'Older adults who experience a decrease in the level of working may be trapped in a self-perpetuating cycle of adverse changes in work and health across the later years' (2013: 813). However, this study focussed on level – retired and part-time and full-time work – and did not examine work characteristics as such.

When looking at transitions to retirement, Zantinge et al. (2015), working in the Netherlands, reviewed changes in smoking, alcohol consumption, physical activity and dietary habits. They found that some studies report an increase in alcohol consumption after retirement, whereas others found a decrease or no change at all, with a causal factor being whether retirement had been chosen or enforced. Studies on changes in smoking and dietary habits, however, were too limited to draw conclusions. Leisure-time physical activity seems to increase slightly after retirement, especially moderately intensive physical activity; however, this increase did not compensate for loss of work-related physical activity, such as the work itself or work-related transportation. They concluded that transitions to retirement are accompanied with both favourable and unfavourable lifestyle changes. Gardiner et al. (2007) found retirement to be the beginning of a period of relative freedom in their study of the redundancy experiences of Welsh steelworkers, following the closure of four steel plants between 2001 and 2003. The older steelworkers who had access to secure pensions talked of their redundancy as being 'a blessing in disguise' in that it led to 'a process of discovery, for the first time in their lives, that they could have control over their time, and exercise choice over whether and when to work' (Gardiner et al., 2007: 486, 85).

Insler (2014) examined the impact of retirement on individuals' health among North American workers, by disentangling simultaneous causal effects. Data from the Health and Retirement Study (HRS) taken biennially between 1992 and 2010 indicated that 'the retirement effect on health is beneficial and significant'. He found that women tend to experience less severe health changes relative to men, while older workers identified as black and Hispanic experience less severe health changes when compared to whites, although here the effect was small. Level of education (as a proxy for wealth in this cohort) was correlated with health preservation.

Investigation into behavioural data, such as smoking and exercise, suggests that retirement may affect health through such channels. With additional leisure time, many retirees practice healthier habits. 'The primary conclusion' based on this data 'is that retirement exerts a beneficial and statistically significant impact on individuals' future health prospects' (2014: 200).

In discussing the mixed findings of previous research, Insler (2014) points to a connection between health insurance access and the decision to work or retire, which may create a spurious link between failing health in retirement. Both Isler in the United States and Vickerstaff (2010) in the United Kingdom observe a survivor effect that can distort an association between ageing, work and health. In other words, uncontrolled surveys of older workers are in danger of assuming a positive relationship between health and work because those who are healthy stay in work and those who are not drop out, rather than workers remaining healthy because they are in work itself.

The notion that working longer will 'add life to longer years' may, then, be of limited value and strike those forced to continue on in low-status, low-paid jobs as "oppressive, irrelevant, or frustrating" (Holstein, 2011: 232). As Holstein explains, there is a difference between returning to work as a white-collar part-time consultant 'and having to work at a minimum wage job just to make ends meet'. For these latter low-paid workers, which includes many women, 'work is often arduous and not a source of self-respect' (2011: 234). McGann et al.'s (2015) group who felt they had no choice but to work were predominantly those in low-pay, low-skill and casualised work. Retirement was seen as a stage of life reserved for 'lucky people' and respondents doubted this would be possible for them; 'they were deeply anxious about the future and described themselves as in a kind of netherworld or limbo between work and retirement' (2015: 4). The people who spend their lives working in physically demanding or psychosocially stressful jobs tend to be those at the bottom of the social gradient in health and have comparatively little time in retirement to reclaim their lives. Policy emphasis given to a looming pension crisis arising from people now having longer, healthier lives, can be amnesic to the fact that gains in health and longevity have been far from universally realised across societies. To take England as an example, average male life expectancy was as high as 88 years in some of the wealthiest parts of London. However, as highlighted by the Marmot Review, life expectancy in the poorest neighbourhoods of England was still only 67 years of age (*Marmot et al., 2010*: 37). And although life-expectancy among all social classes has risen since the 1970s, the gap in life expectancy between lower-skilled workers in manual and heavy physical occupations on the one hand and managers and professionals on the other has actually widened (Phillipson, 2013).

This debate on the positive value of work, as contrasted to the option of a reasonably resourced retirement, has still to encounter a persistent yet puzzling finding: that life satisfaction across the lifecourse follows a 'U' shape for both women and men. In other words things begin well, go into a dive through to the middle years, and begin to rise again between the ages of 55 and 75. Blanchflower and Oswald (2008) maintain that a U-shape in age is found in separate well-being regression equations across 72 developed and developing nations. More recently, it has been observed in the Australian Institute for Family Studies' longitudinal survey data (Qu & de Vaus, 2015) and in the English Longitudinal Study on Ageing (Steptoe, Deaton & Stone, 2015), which concludes: 'These findings suggest that older populations, although less healthy and less productive in general, may be more satisfied with their lives, and experience less stress, worry, and anger than do middle-aged people" (2015: 4).

The dip years, it has to be noted, correspond to the traditional period of working life. Indeed, in terms of attitudes to work, this relationship was first noted by Herzberg et al. in 1957 and then by Clark, Oswald and Warr (1996) and can now be seen to follow a wider trend. That objective and subjective assessments of quality of life diverged in later life had been noted by Cummins (2000) but most surprising of all to labour economists is that happiness does not, in lifecourse terms, appear to be related to wealth and income (Blanchflower & Oswald, 2004). This correspondence between low life satisfaction and working years has yet to be explained.

Work, health and ageing?

It would appear that the best that can be said for existing evidence is that it is mixed. The relationship between work and health appears to depend primarily on job quality and whether people want to work or not work. Working *per se* is not necessarily better for people's health than not working. Neither is it that work benefits older workers and that the relationship between work and health flips from younger to later life. Where opportunities for retirement are available, effects appear to be as much contingent on the quality of the transition as the value of work itself. In addition, claims that work unequivocally benefits people in late life may be a consequence of methodological bias, selective survivorship, and political wishful thinking. The best that can be said is that while work itself may not be healthy, extra years of health do allow for extra years of work.

The commodification of life's time

Combining the changing nature of work, the position of working longer and its effects on health status draws attention to a broader phenomenon, which may not simply question an evaluation of everyday working for older workers but also the changing nature of the lifecourse and the value attributed to the lifetime itself. The tension between work and personal time experienced by many older workers reported in qualitative studies highlights the potential for productive ageing polices to undercut as well as extend agency in later life. And the question needs to be posed of whether there are more subtle costs of extending the lifetime spent at work, on work-life balance and prospects of regaining sovereignty over time. Here, viewing a long life as an opportunity to simply continue working, productivist forms of negotiating increased longevity have become subject to what Beck has described as 'the value imperialism of work' (2000: 7) extended to the experience of later life. Beck (2000) captures how the domain of people's life activity has been increasingly narrowly circumscribed so that 'Everything is work, or else it is nothing' (63). Even leisure and play are now 'negatively imprisoned in the value imperialism of work' in that they are 'imbued with work and its measures of value' (Beck, 2000: 61). In lifecourse terms, policy agendas that ascribe legitimacy to a long life spent in work, convert longevity into economic activity and simultaneously create a commodified economy of time. This reduces the experience of time in later life to its exchange value. A long life thereby becomes subject to 'the subordination of time to the rhythms of the labour market' (Fitzpatrick, 2004: 204), a process that has been intensified by the rise of the flexible economy and postindustrial patterns of work organisation. Just as the organisation of work under capitalism has shaped people's awareness of everyday time in ways that constitute time for personal life existing in the shadow of the time economy of the labour market (Adam, 2003; Noonan, 2009; Svenstrup, 2013), productive ageing agendas exhibit an economy of time that imprisons the experience of time in later life and negatively affects notions of lifetime work-life balance (Biggs et al., 2017). Modes of time utilisation that do not involve either the production or consumption of capital come to be treated as peripheral (Noonan, 2009; Svenstrup, 2013). This gives rise to a restless experience of time that makes it increasingly difficult for people 'to give in' to forms of leisure and play done for their own sake 'without self-contempt and a bad conscience' (Beck, 2000: 61–62).

Noonan (2009), in his essay on the experience of 'surplus' time under capitalism, argues that people's experience and value given to time is shaped, in advanced capitalist economies, by production and consumption and the imperatives of the money-value system. The systems of management regulating people's experience of time spent at work encourages people to experience time as an economic resource not to be wasted (Morello, 1997), which spills over into an experience of time more generally, so that times when 'nothing' happens 'are considered unproductive, wasteful, lost opportunities' (Adam, 2003: 96). Noonan (2009) argues that these governing priorities militate against the potential for self-directed forms of time-utilisation 'by commodifying what people have a mind to do' with any extra time available to them. Spare or surplus (nonwork) time thus comes to be experienced 'as a burden to be filled through some commodified form of activity' (Noonan, 2009: 387). This can be seen in the way surplus time has increasingly come to be associated with activities that involve the consumption of goods or services, such as shopping, going out for coffee or a meal or going to the movies, a concert or the stadium. Indeed, as Himmelweit (1995) observed, decreases in average working hours during the 1950s and 1960s did not so much increase the scope for self-fulfilling activities outside of paid work as result in 'more time for the purchase and consumption of consumer goods'. Noonan's (2009: 387) point is that time that is not in some way work-like provokes 'a restlessness that makes it physically difficult not to be engaged in either production or consumption'.

The restless experience of time has been intensified through the use of Internet technology and globalised time frames, in what Svenstrup has called the 'extensification of work time,' or work-time creep (2013: 16). Not only is the amount of time that people spend working increasing (Lewis, 2003), it no longer obeys fixed chronometric limits as 'all the hours of the day become potential working hours' (Svenstrup, 2013: 15). In other words, paid work is no longer fixed by location or 'working hours' as flexitime and teleworking erode these spatial and temporal boundaries, threatening qualitatively different experiences existing within families or through leisure. While this development was initially greeted with optimism, in so far as it could lead to greater temporal autonomy for workers to balance their working hours around their personal life (Lewis, 2003; Svenstrup, 2013), it has instead paved the way for all time to become potentially production-oriented. These can be expected to have health implications in the immediate term, but also in long-term health consequences for family life, child rearing, diet and exercise, relaxation and recovery time.

The commodification of lifecourse time

The debate on commodification and work-life balance has mostly considered the immediate effects on the value given to time on a day-to-day basis. However, traces of the lack of rest that Noonan and others observe are also evident in societal responses to the increased potential afforded by a long life. The 'positive' images of ageing portrayed within contemporary policy revolve around modes of time use that encourage later life to be appreciated principally for its exchange value through work or work-like activities such as volunteering, plus 'active consumer lifestyles' (Featherstone & Hepworth, 1995: 44) and in resisting structured dependency by 'joining in this shopping trip' (Gilleard, 1996: 495).

Here, commodification of the lifecourse can be populated by both productive and consumption-based activities, each of which fills otherwise 'empty' space. Activities that differentiate distinctive phases of life become eclipsed by an expanded period of 'active middle age', which has, particularly in the realm of policy, shifted into later life being claimed by 'the value imperialism of work'. This occurs both as a greater proportion of the lifecourse becomes production oriented and through the structured consumption of the commodities produced. The value of the 'surplus' time afforded by gains in longevity thus comes to be appreciated for its exchange value and, as Adam says about everyday time, 'a commodity that we can use, allocate, control and exchange on the labour market' (2003: 98). Little is asked about how a long life has otherwise been used by a majority who have hitherto been able to find healthy fulfilment through retirement. But as Adam argues, once time comes to be experienced as an economic resource not to be wasted, 'any time that cannot be accorded a money value is consequently suspect and held in low-esteem' (2003: 117). Thus, according to Bass (2002), 'Personal enrichment is not included' and 'meditation, religious reflection, personal growth, reminiscence . . . and education for expressive purposes are all outside the definition of productive ageing' (Bass, 2002).

The commodification of the lifetime arises through but is also driving a way of attributing value to a long life that fills it with work and work-like activity. This occurs both quantitatively, in the colonisation of the extra time people have to live, and qualitatively, by filling up those extra years and in driving out other forms of meaningful activity. Unfortunately, this narrative structure can also be detected in debates on health that wish to replace chronological with functional age (WHO, 2002). At first encounter, functional age, a marker for ageing based on what a person can do rather than the age he or she has reached, appears to make sense as a means of calibrating vulnerability and need. However, as work and health have become increasingly associated, the interconnection between productive ageing and functional ageing becomes blurred (see also Chapter 7). Functionality becomes the bodily signifier of productivity, itself an agent of commodification and a translation of intrinsic value into extrinsic, use value.

The UK Commission of Employment and Skills' (2014) report on workplace needs in 2030 provides scenarios that exacerbate rather than mitigate the trends noted earlier. Scarcity and competition for work would also increase as robotics strip out further layers of both routine and professional employment (World Economic Forum, 2016). This has led some authors to argue for a citizen wage and 'a high-tec future free from work' (Smircek & Williams, 2015). However, policy discourse on adult ageing shows little sign of valuing longevity other than an increase in commodification through work. Official policy discourses and uncritical gerontologies paint the prospect of delayed retirement in highly optimistic terms, as a welcome alternative to the structured dependency of the welfare state. However, evidence on the health and wider social goods associated with the extension of working life is at best ambivalent. The costs on the lifecourse-based work-life balance and reduced prospects of regaining sovereignty over time might only be expected to exacerbate trends that challenge mental and physical well-being. Trends towards increased precarity in later life, generated by restricted pension access and uncertain working conditions, must be placed against those that provide improved workplace conditions for older workers and reduce social ageism. It is nevertheless easy to mistake increased work as a solution to ageist practices, where, when the health benefits and deficits are taken into account, they may prove to be the reverse.

Concluding comments

These two chapters, on the relationship between work and ageing, began by trying to make sense of a debate that proposed a particular solution to the purpose of a long life in the context of adaptation to a more balanced generational demographic. Regardless of its stability as a foundation for an inclusive longevity, work has become a defining marker for social value and the principal container for notions of activity and engagement in later life. The medium through which this took place has been predominantly social policy, which has increasingly come to colonise debates on health and its relation to growing older with the need to extend working life. When the evidence is assessed, a causal connection between these two is by no means clear and begins to look like a form of political wishful thinking. It reverses the logic of the work-health association, in the service of priorities arising from elsewhere. The most that can be said of the relationship is that a healthy, long life allows people to work longer but not that working longer keeps people healthy.

The extension of work-thinking into other parts of the lifecourse, called here the commodification of life's time, adds a new critical dimension to this colonisation. Lifetime commodification supplies one mechanism at play in evacuating alternative life priorities with which to engage the gift of healthy extra years.

A dynamic of denial, hypothesised for this form of policy discourse, exists at a number of different levels. First, it enhances a guiding myth of agelessness, which is closely related to notions of workplace-based activity and productive engagement. It is, in other words, productiveness or functional capacity that determines legitimacy and not age. Second, empirical evidence on the health value of alternatives to work, such as adequately funded retirement, have largely been sidelined as an inconvenient truth. Third, different age-based priorities, arising from a changed lifecourse, have been eclipsed, only being accepted if they conform to the dominant narrative.

In sum, it appears that there is no single policy panacea when it comes to work as an answer to a long life or as a means of addressing generational distinctiveness. Cooperation and competition between generations is addressed in Chapter 10. Here we have seen that older workers both want and don't want to continue working. This depends upon the quality of work available and the life circumstances of the people involved. Similarly, there is evidence that both retirement and continued working can have positive health consequences, although it is safer to say that healthy ageing creates the possibility of a longer working life rather than work enhancing health. Work, it appears, emerges as the dominant way in which activity is legitimised in midlife and beyond, by eschewing positive discontinuity and positive othering. A work mentality has colonised wide areas of everyday living largely overwhelming lifetime with present-centred thinking. Through the colonisation of life's time itself, productive and active ageing have edged into areas of the lifecourse that had previously allowed for personal and social autonomy.

References

Adam, B. (2003, December). When time is money: Contested rationalities of time in the theory and practice of work. *Theoria, 102,* 94–125.

The Australian Psychological Society. (2002). *Psychology and ageing: A position paper prepared for the Australian psychological society.* Melbourne: APS.

Bass, S. A. (2002). Productive aging. In D. J. Ekerdt (Ed.), *Encyclopedia of aging* (pp. 1130–1132). Ann Arbor: University of Michigan, Macmillan Reference.

Bass, S. A., Caro, F. J., & Chen, Y. P. (1993). *Achieving a productive aging society.* Westport, CT: Auburn House.

Beck, U. (2000). *The brave new world of work.* Cambridge, England: Polity Press.

Beynon, H. (1984). *Working for ford.* London, England: Penguin Books.

Biggs, S., McGann, M., Bowman, D., & Kimberley, H. (2017). Work, health and the commodification of life's time: Reframing work–life balance and the promise of a long life. *Ageing and Society, 37*(7), 1458–1483.

Blanchflower, D. G., & Oswald, A. J. (2004). Well-being over time in Britain and the USA. *Journal of Public Economics, 88*(7), 1359–1386.

Blanchflower, D. G., & Oswald, A. J. (2008). Is well-being U-shaped over the life cycle? *Social Science & Medicine, 66*(8), 1733–1749.

Brinkley, I., Fauth, R., Mahdon, M., & Theodoropoulou, S. (2010). Is knowledge work better for us? Knowledge workers, good work, and well-being. London: The Work Foundation. DOI:10.13140/RG.2.1.1649.8720

Butler, R. N., & Gleason, H. P. (1985). *Productive aging*. New York, NY: Springer Publishing Company.

Butler, R. N., Miller, R. A., Perry, D., Carnes, B. A., Williams, T. F., Cassel, C., & Martin, G. M. (2008). New model of health promotion and disease prevention for the 21st century. *British Medical Journal, 337*, 149–150.

Calasanti, T., & King, N. (2011). A feminist lens on the third age: Refining the framework. In D. C. Carr & Kathrin S. Komp (Eds.), *Gerontology in the era of the third age* (pp. 67–85). New York, NY: Springer Publishing Company.

Clark, A., Oswald, A., & Warr, P. (1996). Is job satisfaction U-shaped in age? *Journal of Occupational and Organizational Psychology, 69*(1), 57–81.

Commission of the European Communities. (1999). *Towards a Europe for all ages: Promoting prosperity and intergenerational solidarity*. Commission of the European Communities. Retrieved from http://ec.europa.eu/employment_social/social_situation/docs/com221_en.pdf

Cummins, R. A. (2000). Objective and subjective quality of life: An interactive model. *Social Indicators Research, 52*, 52–72.

EIP-AHA. (2012). European innovation partnership on active and healthy ageing: Action plan on innovation for age-friendly buildings, cities & environments. Retrieved September 25, 2015, from https://ec.europa.eu/research/innovation-union/pdf/active-healthy-ageing/d4_action_plan.pdf

Ekerdt, D. J. (2010). Frontiers of research on work and retirement. *Journal of Gerontology: Social Sciences, 65*(1), 69–80.

European Union. (2012). European year of active ageing & intergenerational solidarity 2012. Retrieved May 8, 2017, from www.age-platform.eu/images/stories/EY2012_Campaign.pdf

Featherstone, M., & Hepworth, M. (1995). Images of positive ageing. In M. Featherstone & A. Wernick (Eds.), *Images of ageing* (pp. 29–47). London, England: Routledge.

Field, J., Burke, R. J., & Cooper, C. L. (Eds.). (2013). *The sage handbook of aging, work and society*. London, England: Sage.

Fitzpatrick, T. (2004). Social policy and time. *Time & Society, 13*(2–3), 197–219.

Gardiner, J., Stuart, M., Forde, C., Greenwood, I., MacKenzie, R., & Perrett, R. (2007). Work–life balance and older workers: Employees' perspectives on retirement transitions following redundancy. *The International Journal of Human Resource Management, 18*(3), 476–489.

Gilleard, C. (1996). Consumption and identity in later life. *Ageing and Society, 16*(2), 489–498.

Herzberg, F., Mausnes, B., Peterson, R. O., & Capwell, D. F. (1957). *Job attitudes: Review of research and opinion*. Pittsburgh, PA: Psychological Service of Pittsburgh.

Himmelweit, S. (1995). The discovery of "unpaid work": The social consequences of the expansion of "work". *Feminist Economics, 1*(2), 1–19.

Holstein, M. (2011). Cultural ideals, ethics, and agelessness: A critical perspective on the third age. In D. C. Carr & K. Komp (Eds.), *Gerontology in the era of the third age* (pp. 225–242). New York, NY: Springer Publishing Company.

Insler, M. (2014). The health consequences of retirement. *Journal of Human Resources Winter, 49*(1), 195–233.

Johnson, K. J., & Mutchler, J. E. (2014). The emergence of a positive gerontology: From disengagement to social involvement. *The Gerontologist, 54*, 93–100.

Lain, D. (2012). Working past 65 in the UK and the USA: Segregation into "Lopaq" occupations? *Work, Employment and Society, 26*(1), 78–94.

Lewis, J. (2003). Economic citizenship: A comment. *Social Politics: International Studies in Gender, State & Society, 10*(2), 176–185.

Loretto, W., Lain, D., & Vickerstaff, S. (2013). Guest editorial: Rethinking retirement: Changing realities for older workers and employee relations? *Employee Relations, 35*(3), 248–256.

Marmot, M. G., Allen, J., Goldblatt, P., Boyce, T., McNeish, D., Grady, M., & Geddes, I. (2010). *Fair society, healthy lives: Strategic review of health inequalities in England post-2010.* London, England: UK Government.

Marmot, M. G., Ryff, C. D., Bumpass, L. L., Shipley, M., & Marks, N. F. (1997). Social inequalities in health: Next questions and converging evidence. *Social Science & Medicine, 44*(6), 901–910.

McGann, M., Bowman, D., Kimberley, H., & Biggs, S. (2015). *Too old to work, too young to retire.* Research Insight Report. Melbourne: Brotherhood of St Laurence.

Miller, R. (2009). "Dividends" from research on aging: Can biogerontologists, at long last, find something useful to do? *Journals of Gerontology, Series A: Biological Sciences and Medical Sciences, 64*(2), 157–160.

Morello, G. (1997). Sicilian time. *Time & Society, 6*(1), 55–69.

Noonan, J. (2009). Free time as a necessary condition of free life. *Contemporary Political Theory, 8*(4), 377–393.

OECD. (1998). *Maintaining prosperity in an ageing society: The OECD study on the policy implications of ageing.* France: Organisation for Economic Cooperation and Development.

Olshansky, J., Beard, J., & Börsch-Supan, A. (2012). The longevity dividend: Health as an investment. In J. Beard, S. Biggs, D. E. Bloom, L. P. Fried, P. Hogan, A. Kalache & S. J. Olshansky (Eds.), *Global population ageing: Peril or promise?* (pp. 57–60). Geneva, Switzerland: World Economic Forum.

Olshansky, S. J., Perry, D., Miller, R. A., & Butler, R. N. (2006). In pursuit of the longevity dividend. *The Scientist, 20*(3), 28–36.

Phillipson, C. (1998). *Reconstructing old age: New agendas in social theory and practice.* London, England: Sage.

Phillipson, C. (2013). *Ageing.* New Jersey: John Wiley & Sons.

Qu, L., & de Vaus, A. (2015). *Life satisfaction across life course transitions: Australian family trends* (No. 8). Melbourne: Australian Institute of Family Studies.

Rowe, J. W., & Kahn, R. L. (1997). Successful aging. *The Gerontologist, 37*(4), 433–440.

Sahlgren, G. H. (2013). *Work longer, live healthier: The relationship between economic activity, health and government policy.* London, England: Institute of Economic Affairs.

Siegrist, J., & Wahrendorf, M. (2009). Participation in socially productive activities and quality of life in early old age: Findings from SHARE. *Journal of European Social Policy, 19*(4), 317–326.

Siegrist, J., & Wahrendorf, M. (2013). Quality of work, wellbeing, and retirement. In J. Field, R. J. Burke & C. L. Cooper (Eds.), *The sage handbook of aging, work and society* (pp. 314–326). London, England: Sage.

Smircek, N., & Williams, A. (2015). *Inventing the future: Postcapitalism and a world without work.* New York, NY: Verso Books.

Steptoe, A., Deaton, A., & Stone, A. A. (2015). Subjective wellbeing, health, and ageing. *The Lancet, 385*(9968), 640–648.

Svenstrup, M. (2013). Towards a new time culture: Conceptual and perceptual tools. Retrieved October 1, 2015, from http://time-culture.net/

Taylor, P. (2010). Cross national trends in work and retirement. In C. Phillipson & D. Dannefer (Eds.), *Handbook of social gerontology* (pp. 540–548). London, England: Sage.

Trades Union Congress. (2012). Half a million people approaching state pension age are too ill to work. Retrieved October 1, 2015, from www.tuc.org.uk/economic-issues/pensions-and-retirement/half-million-people-approaching-state-pension-age-are-too

Tuomi, K., Huuhtanen, P., Nykyri, E., & Ilmarinen, J. (2001). Promotion of work ability, the quality of work and retirement. *Occupational Medicine, 51*(5), 318–324.

The UK Commission of Employment and Skills. (2014). The future of work jobs and skills in 2030. Retrieved from www.gov.uk/government/uploads/system/uploads/attachment_data/file/303334/er84-the-future-of-work-evidence-report.pdf

Vaughan-Jones, H., & Barham, L. (2009). *Healthy work: Challenges and opportunities to 2030.* London, England: British United Provident Association.

Vickerstaff, S. (2010). Older workers: The "unavoidable obligation" of extending our working lives? *Sociology Compass, 4*(10), 869–879.

Victor, C. R. (1991). *Health and health care in later life.* Buckingham: Open University Press.

Von Bonsdorff, M. E., Shultz, K. S., Leskinen, E., & Tansky, J. (2009). The choice between retirement and bridge employment: A continuity theory and life course perspective. *The International Journal of Aging and Human Development, 69*(2), 79–100.

Wahrendorf, M., Blane, D., Matthews, K., & Siegrist, J. (2015). Linking quality of work in midlife to volunteering during retirement: A European study. *Journal of Population Ageing, 9*(1–2), 113–130.

Warr, P. (1997). Age, work, and mental health. In K. W. Schaie & C. Schooler (Eds.), *The impact of work on older adults* (pp. 252–296). New York, NY: Springer Publishing Company.

Warr, P. (2007). *Work, happiness, and unhappiness.* New York, NY: Laurence Erlbaum.

Warr, P. B., & Wall, T. D. (1975). *Work and well-being* (Vol. 578). London, England: Penguin Books.

Westerlund, H., Kivimäki, M., Singh-Manoux, A., Melchior, M., Ferrie, J. E., Pentti, J., . . . Vahtera, J. (2009). Self-rated health before and after retirement in France (GAZEL): A cohort study. *The Lancet, 374*(9705), 1889–1896.

Westerlund, H., Kivimäki, M., Singh-Manoux, A., Melchior, M., Ferrie, J. E., Pentti, J., . . . Vahtera, J. (2010). Effect of retirement on major chronic conditions and fatigue: French GAZEL occupational cohort study. *British Medical Journal, 341*, c6149.

Wickrama, K. A. S., O'Neal, C. W., Kwag, K. H., & Lee, T. K. (2013). Is working later in life good or bad for health? An investigation of multiple health outcomes. *Journals of Gerontology: Psychological Sciences and Social Sciences, 68*(5), 807–815.

Winefield, A. H. (2000). Stress in academe: Some recent research findings. In D. T. Kenny, J. G. Carlson, F. J. McGuigan & J. L. Sheppard (Eds.), *Stress and health* (pp. 437–446). Amsterdam: Harwood Academic Publishers.

World Economic Forum. (2016). The future of jobs: Employment, skills and workforce strategy for the fourth industrial revolution. Retrieved from www3.weforum.org/docs/WEF_Future_of_Jobs.pdf

World Health Organization. (2002). Active ageing: a policy framework. Second World Assembly on Aging. Madrid, Spain: World Health Organization.

Zantinge, E. M., van den Berg, M., Smit, H. A., & Picavet, H. S. J. (2015). Retirement and a healthy lifestyle: Opportunity or pitfall? A narrative review of the literature. *European Journal of Public Health, 24*(3), 433–439.

5   Spirit, belief and the in-between

Key themes

- Adult ageing has been associated with increasing spirituality
- Spirituality draws attention to liminal or in-between experiences
- There is some evidence of the positive effects of belief
- Negotiating vulnerability is a distinctive narrative on ageing
- While adult ageing can be discontinuous, the soul is perceived to be continuous
- Emphasis is placed on transcending rather than avoiding difficulty and finitude
- Different belief systems offer universalising yet distinctive perspectives on ageing

Spirituality, belief and ageing

A discussion on the relationship between ageing and the life of the spirit proposes a different set of questions to the materiality of the body through health and labour economics. To many readers in secular societies, its idiom can be both strange and disconnected from their everyday lives. As Coleman (2011) points out, however, this is by no means a universal phenomenon, with many parts of the world experiencing an increase in both spirituality and religious participation. In China, the postcommunist world, and in Africa a variety of forms of Christianity have experienced rapid expansion (Coleman et al., 2011), while Islam, Hinduism and Buddhism have continued to attract believers (Coleman, Begum & Jaleel, 2011). As an academic discipline, the gerontology of religion and spirituality has a continuing presence, particularly in North America (Atchley, 2009; Nelson-Becker, 2017). The questions that spiritual life sets for adult ageing mean that personal and social priorities cease to make sense in the same way as they do within materialist narratives. Adoption of a spiritual belief system can involve putting oneself in the hands of a higher power bigger than the self, and in touch with priorities that are beyond immediate physical concerns. One is placed in a liminal, or in-between, state concerning both realities, with belief exerting influence in the role of a gate-keeper to aspects of human experience that go beyond the everyday.

Liminality is an important concept for discourses of the spirit. As a word, *liminal* has its roots in Latin, meaning to be on a threshold, and has come to represent the state of being between two different realities. These realities can refer to states of mind or a point of connection between alternate worlds and therefore comes to contain the tensions between these realities. When one finds oneself in a liminal state, the barrier between realities is experienced as being particularly thin, and the distinction between everyday experience and an alternative form of being is said to become transparent as the two are interconnected. For a believer, this places the everyday in touch with the sublime. As a result, one ends up interrogating the lifecourse, intergenerational relations and purpose of a long life in a particular way. It offers a different frame of reference on the body, work and forms of interpersonal conduct to that supplied by economics or medicine.

Making a distinction between spirituality and religious practices has been a point of contention in this literature, with Coleman (2011) opting for a more inclusive label of belief. He defines this as 'a belief in a transcendent reality usually filled with supernatural beings with which communication, connection and even identification or co-inherence is possible' (2011: 5).

Writers have struggled with this trio, and belief, while an overarching category, also includes a series of shorthands that people use to navigate their worlds, which may or may not have a liminal connection. It would also include materialist philosophies, such as Marxism and humanism, which specifically exclude religious belief systems (Wilkinson & Coleman, 2011). In a phenomenal sense, in the sense in which such realities are experienced in daily life, believers may make few explicit distinctions between religious belief and spirituality in so far as one becomes the medium through which the other is expressed. The most commonly made division between the two is to distinguish institutional structures and practices from personal experiences (Koenig, McCullough & Larson, 2001; Ridge et al., 2008). Religion can be observed, attendance measured, and rituals and symbols categorised. Both MacKinlay (2001) and Coleman (2011) regret the fact that discussion of religious practice has often deadened debate, being more easily measured than subjective beliefs. Sadler, Biggs and Glaser (2013) found that some older adults had difficulty with the concept of an independent spirituality, mostly because they considered the term to be abstract and hard to pin down or because they saw it as part of a relationship between the self and God or nature. Elsewhere spirituality has been defined as reflecting 'beliefs and values pertaining to the personal search for meaning and purpose in or beyond life' (Sadler & Biggs, 2006), where spirituality is seen as a broader construct than religion and that individuals' spiritual perspectives may or may not be shaped within an institutionalised religious context. In Sadler et al.'s (2013) study, non-religious elders often claimed to experience spiritual feelings through music, art, relationships and a sense of connection to the universe.

The issues that are the focus of this chapter are less about established religious bodies and have a greater concern with the understandings, philosophies and consequences that such beliefs can have for later life and intergenerational relations. In many ways, spiritual belief, for which the word *belief* will be used interchangeably within this chapter, has the goal of answering the 'why' question of life's purpose and thus, for the current inquiry, promises to discover what is said about the 'purpose of a long life'.

Why questions

'Why' questions occur at certain points in the lifecourse:

> The first is age 3–4 years, when 'why' is the beginning of logic in a child's development. The second is adolescence. 'Why should I or shouldn't I?' Much of this is a search for personal identity, that is 'Who am I?' The third is in the face of adversity, particularly serious illness, 'Why me?'
>
> (Flynn, personal communication, 2015)

And while illness can make older people re-categorise themselves as 'old', ageing has also become associated with death and decline (Biggs, 1999). Flynn continues that 'Why' implies going beyond 'how' in the same way as a family who asks, 'Why is my house flooded?' are not particularly helped by an explanation of weather fronts.

Cole (1992) has argued that spiritual belief constitutes an awakening of cultural resources to respond to existential issues, vulnerability and dependencies that ageing brings to the fore. And within a sometimes either aggressively anti- or intolerantly religious social climate, we can ask the extent to which spirituality composes an alternative behind the masquerade of ageing. In terms of purpose and age, the degree to which spiritual beliefs provide a roadmap to self-development and relationships with others may simply have been eclipsed by more pressingly incomplete answers. These may be 'how' answers arising from medical practice or 'what' answers pressing greater consumerism or productivity. From a spiritual perspective, it appears as if questions about the means to a long life and how to fill it have been substituted for the purpose.

To what degree, then, would a focus on the spirit propose a solution for cultural adaptation of which ageing in itself and ageing in relationship to others are key components? What sort of answer would it give to the question of 'Why a long life?'

Are belief and spirit good for you?

While spiritual belief is a complex and multifaceted construct, there are certain common assumptions in the literature about its status as a universal human characteristic. Moberg (2001), for example speaks of an 'awareness of the hunger for eternity that seems implanted in the human heart' (2001: 230), while Atchley (2009) describes it as encompassing "beliefs, practices, and experiences that loosely revolve around an inner domain of human experience" (2009: 2). Hays and Hays (2003), speaking of Christian belief, argue that at least in terms of universality, 'nowhere is growing old itself described as a problem' and 'is on the side of similarity rather than difference between aged and young' (2003: 17).

When it comes to the process of ageing, a variety of responses can be seen in the literature. Moody (1997) and Moberg (2001) both indicate, using census and longitudinal studies, that Americans engage in higher levels of spirituality, prayer and religious observance as they grow older. However, Kaufmann (2010) has argued that religious observance shows few age patterns. The trend is compounded, in this Western European context, by lower levels of formal religious involvement among older adults and in the general population than in the United States. Studies largely based on North American survey data have found gender and ethnic group differences in the importance of religious beliefs and practices, with older women and those from black and ethnic minority groups reporting higher levels of both (Chatters et al., 2009; Taylor, Chatters & Jackson, 2007). These findings were supported in Sadler et al.'s (2013) British study. Here, Black Caribbean older men and women in particular defined spirituality in terms of belief in and relationship with a transcendent God. Similar definitions of spirituality among older African Americans were found by Cohen, Thomas and Williamson (2008), whose respondents viewed God as a benevolent influence, supporting believers through oppression, 'daily struggles and difficult times'.

Some research has been undertaken on whether spiritual belief is good for you. A number of studies have reported positive links between spirituality, health and well-being in later life (Moberg, 2001; Kirby, Coleman & Daley, 2004; Koenig et al., 2001; Zimmer et al., 2016). These have included increased personal rather than externally motivated sources of self-worth and greater self-confidence, plus an ability to put aside past resentments and disappointments. Wink and Dillon (2008) found that religiousness was positively related, in late adulthood, to well-being arising from positive relations with others, social and community engagement and concern for younger generations. Spirituality was positively related to personal growth, creativity, and knowledge-building. Neither was associated with narcissism. There is also evidence that spiritual and religious beliefs can contribute to successful coping with chronic illness in later life (Harvey & Silverman, 2007). MacKinlay (2001) speaks of spiritual themes arising during in-depth interviews with older people, including self-sufficiency/vulnerability, wisdom/final meanings, relationship/isolation, and hope/fear, plus as a response to ultimate (final) meaning in life. Atchley (2009) reports qualities identified by older research participants to include stillness, peace, mystery, clarity of seeing, meaning, universal love in the face of suffering, connection with the ground of being, wonder, trust, transformation, call to serve, and desire to pursue a spiritual journey. Yet despite these confirming features, research evidence on spiritual belief is limited when compared to other elements of adult ageing. One can feel the frustration in Coleman's observation, writing in 2011, that while

> we have learned so much in the last half century about the biological, social and psychological processes involved in human ageing . . . we have neglected the spiritual dimension. This neglect is even more surprising when one takes into account that the later stages of life raise fundamental questions about the purpose and meaning of life.
>
> (2011: 1)

When harnessed to post-enlightenment's suspicion of superstition and a humanist rejection of the divine, contemporary secular society can leave the profession of spiritual belief appearing naïve, if not absurd. However, those who have studied the relationship between ageing and spirit have come to a very different conclusion. Coleman, drawing on data from the Southampton longitudinal study (2011), maintains that 'life is unimaginable without belief . . . to act is to be purposeful and beliefs give us purpose . . . beliefs are common and an essential part of ordinary living . . . (and) . . . a source of guidance in the choice of goals and decisions that we make' (2011: 2).

'If we feel our lives are not giving us what we want,' says Moody (1997), 'and if we suspect we're headed down a dead end street, then we have to ask ourselves what we can do to make things better' (1997: 31). One can do nothing, he claims, and accept the consequences of living the same way as in the past or seek a spiritually informed way out.

Vulnerability

So what are the questions that spiritual belief addresses that alternative explanations of age and purpose find so hard to fulfil?

One of the key issues facing adults as they grow older, and one that is increasingly exercising the minds of policy makers and planners as well as people living a long life, is the question of vulnerability. Vulnerability can be expensive to fix and inhibits social engagement, yet is perhaps a core aspect of being human. It is also a quality that a number of writers claim has been pushed out from everyday experience in the public sphere. A rejection of vulnerability has been linked to a 'post-dependency culture' that fragments experience between strength and weakness, being reflected back to us in fragmented service systems (Dartington, 2010). Such cultures harbour, it is argued, a malignancy of thought towards dependence (Davenhill, 2008) and a denial of loss (Holstein et al., 2010). As part of this process, our everyday interdependence on one another would be replaced by 'normal invulnerability' (Baars, 2012) in our conduct, in everyday life, at work, and in public institutions. This rejection of vulnerability would contribute to an othering process aimed at those who have little choice except to be vulnerable. And while this is accepted as a necessary process in the development of children as they emerge into a less-dependent state, the age-other comes to contain adult vulnerability, including the potential threats to identity that such a state might hold for the not yet old. It contains what we have no desire to be.

In spite of this cultural aversion to vulnerability in the toughened up, independent worlds of the public sphere, Baars (2012) argues that it should be recognised as an essential part of the human situation, existing as a continuum in everyday life and becoming increasingly important as we grow older. He goes further in suggesting that vulnerability holds the promise of a common bond between self and other, including the age-other:

> A sense of possible harm is indispensable for responsible actions and to face the possible and ultimately inevitable death of others and ourselves, may contribute to a fuller experience of the value of a relationship . . . Sensitivity for vulnerability is to an important degree constitutive of the quality of the inter-human condition, and shapes how and with what intensity we take part in life.
>
> (Baars, 2012: 204)

When one is vulnerable, or is suffering, the way that this races to the top of our priorities potentiates an empathic understanding of others in a similar position. Singer (1991), a Utilitarian philosopher, gives sensitivity to suffering a central role in our ability to recognise the universal nature of human identity. It bridges the gap between self and other. The

> suffering of another being is very similar to my own suffering and . . . matters just as much to that other being as my own suffering matters to me . . . from this perspective we can see that our own sufferings and pleasures are very like the sufferings and pleasures of others, just because they are 'other'. This remains true whatever way 'otherness' is defined, as long as the capacity for suffering or pleasure remains.
>
> (1991: 264)

Singer quotes with approval a union activist, Henry Spira, who continued to pursue causes in later life wherever he could 'do the most to reduce the universe of pain and suffering'. While no friend of religiosity, Singer believes an ability in certain people to 'take the view of the universe', and step beyond their own immediate concerns, is key to a moral life and in bridging the gap between the narrow pursuit of self-interest and collective benevolence.

As we grow older, and particularly as we enter a fourth age of increasing physical and mental frailty, vulnerability can become a constitutive part of daily life. Both Holstein et al. (2010) and Grenier and Phillison (2014) maintain that an understanding of autonomy in old age needs to incorporate loss and dependency if it is to take account of 'the kinds of selves we are, or are struggling to be, when loss impedes what might otherwise be taken for granted' (2014: 256). However, a focus on vulnerability is not without its critics. Tornstam (2005), the author of *Gerotranscendence*, derides what he calls 'the misery perspective' that he sees in the concerns of mainstream gerontology. According to Tornstam, an overconcern for ill health and social injustice paints a negative picture of the potential inherent in old age, feeding a need to perceive elders as feeble and weak 'in order for us to feel sorry for them . . . and solve the problem of our contempt for unproductive, ineffective and dependent older people' (2005: 13). However, this analysis suggests no mechanisms for explaining how such a rejection operates, the realities of social and bodily forms of disadvantage in later life and the processes of othering that follow from it. Gerotranscendence has been associated with spirituality (Sadler and Biggs, 201), however, and gerontologists studying spiritual belief have taken a different view, seeing a sensitivity to vulnerability in oneself and in others as a key component of a spiritual long life. Suffering has been closely connected to transcendence by the existential philosopher and psychotherapist Victor Frankl (1955), a concentration camp survivor, who valued learning to transcend difficulty, rather than trying to avoid it. Frankl speaks of a need to nurture a process of 'forgetting self' that enables a person to survive through any suffering and rise beyond it.

Both Coleman and MacKinlay report that belief assists older adults to transcend the vulnerability that accompanies old age. Coleman (2011) notes the capacity religious belief can implant to 'endure hardship and remain resolute in the pursuit of goals' and maintains that older adults in the Southampton study report beliefs that support them in understanding and coping with life's challenges. Vulnerability is, according to MacKinlay (2014), largely outside of individual control in the here and now but also in possible future events, such as dementia or physical frailty. She reports that her respondents, living in the community and in residential care, cope by drawing on their beliefs to move from doing to being, in the sense that increasing decrements and an inability to do past activities can be overcome through adopting a transcendent position. Whilst a little vague, this process appears to reflect both a greater in-touchness with immediate experience combined with an awareness of the universal, yet passing nature of suffering that accompanies frail old age. Dartington (2010), drawing on his experience as an organisational consultant and as a carer for a loved one living with dementia, argues that recognising personal and interpersonal dependence leads to a rediscovery of the 'human element' and that 'there are other ways of managing anxiety in our world, including the institutional structures that give us some security,' which can provide a 'respect for the vulnerability in others that we seek to deny in ourselves' (2010: 29). He sees lack of personal control as a challenge to a dominating phantasy of presumed omnipotence that runs through everyday working and institutional life. An awareness of vulnerability counteracts these feelings by opening an individuals' 'capacity for attachment, trust, reliance on others, as well as self-reliance' (2010: 43).

While neither Baars nor Dartington favour a spiritual solution to the questions raised by vulnerability and dependence, they agree that a growing awareness of them, in self and in others, is a universal human phenomenon that is often suppressed in order to cope with the demands of daily existence. It may even be possible to draw the conclusion that vulnerability potentiates a connective motivation – that we are all, so to speak, in the same corporeal boat. There is also an intuition, running through the debate on vulnerability that it is not a fixed state, but rather an intimation of in-betweeness and transition. The persons concerned are caught in the process of liminal dislocation, where previous certainties no longer hold and a new understanding of their place in the human lifecourse is called into play.

This discourse positions belief in relation to material vicissitudes of the ageing body and in many ways places transcendence alongside the work of Baltes and his associates (1999, 2005) as a coping strategy to compensate for the negative effects of ageing. A second theme can be identified that draws attention to the role of belief in addressing a sense of longing, lack or dread. These feelings accompany an increasing awareness of ageing as a period of decline but again point to a more common human experience.

Lack and suffering

A feeling of emptiness has been recognised by existential and humanist philosophers in boredom, apathy and a sense of despair (Cooper, 2017) and in psychotherapy has been labelled a 'nameless dread' (Bion, 1962), an underlying fear of annihilation that most of us manage to fend off most of the time but can force itself into consciousness in times of melancholy, reflection and vulnerability. According to Bion, people continually manage their relationship with the world in order to avoid such feelings of hopelessness.

The incompleteness heralded by such feelings gives spirituality both its symptom and its cure. Moody (1997) reports that his workshop participants have experienced 'a primal pain of separation that we all feel – a separation from something deep in our hearts and souls' . . . concluding that 'We're all in a state of mourning for something we've lost' (1997: 27).

Within the Abramic religious tradition, this sense of incompleteness and existential pain is interpreted as an intimation of our separation from God. It can be traced from the fall of Adam and Eve through to the world's rejection of Jesus Christ, who embodied the healing integration of God and humanity. It is also a strong theme in Hindu and Buddhist traditions, where particular attention has been paid to the transience of things.

In their short article 'Self and suffering, a Buddhist-Christian conversation', Ingram and Loy (2005) propose that 'all life forms suffer – including human beings – just because they are alive' (99). This form of natural suffering 'just is' and presents a different set of issues to the suffering imposed by other humans. From a Christian perspective, the problem is that we are estranged from each other whilst living our lives as if we are the centre of the universe. We are not necessarily in control of such forces, but they are nevertheless of our collective making and create a separation from God and from others. This separation is fundamentally unbearable, and indeed is, within the Lutheran tradition, a definition of a sinful state. Sin, then, is the pain of separation from God. Rather than the pursuit of subjective aims, this sense of lack will only be extinguished as we get back into synchrony with God's 'initial aim for the self'; the life of Jesus is the most perfect example of a personal will dissolved in the will of God. Vulnerability and suffering, encapsulated in a sense of lack and incompletion, then, point human beings to 'the fundamental character of existence: from great suffering for all life, including God, something other than suffering emerges that is redemptive . . . but pain and suffering is still pain and suffering . . . inherent within life itself' (102). According to this view, the route out of despair runs through compassion for others and care for the community and the weak, because these activities are pleasing to and bring us closer to God. Vulnerability and our actions to remedy it, especially in others, create a liminal state where we are more in touch with being between material and spiritual worlds.

In the Buddhist tradition, suffering is characterised by 'dukkha', of which there are three types. The first form of suffering consists of physical, mental and emotional pain prompted by impermanence. Because each individual experience is going to end, it acts as an intimation of death, which then casts a shadow over every pleasure we experience. Nothing in the material world is reliable. The second form arises from an attachment to selfhood, which is seen as an accumulation of habits of feeling, thinking and acting. Each of these is a conditioned state and again is transient. Finally, ignorance and craving stick us to a material and impermanent world; we crave sensations from which only the practice of mindfulness can release us. In summary, all of these phenomena are constructed on transience and remind us of our 'sense of *lack* – that is the sense that something is missing in our lives, that something is *wrong* with us' (Ingram and Loy, 2005: 103). All forms of activity, consumption and engagement with the material world are deflections away from this emptiness, while, at the same time, attachment to them is its cause. And here there are close parallels to Christian thinking in so far as 'the emptiness that has always been present is now revealed in stark nakedness, no longer hidden by the social and psychological props that society has taken away . . . yet transforms into . . . a sacramental process of emptying', in order to lead one to God, 'an emptiness that signifies an inward and spiritual grace at the core' (MacKinlay, 2001: 61).

As Sapp (2010) points out, for all the major religious traditions, ageing is connected to coming to terms with mortality and, in this sense, transience and liminality. Hays and Hays (2003) suggest that the matter of greatest concern to be found in religious texts is the trajectory towards mortality, rather than the ageing process itself, such that 'those who trust in God are not locked into the past, neither into traditional social roles nor into well-worn paths chosen in earlier life' and the religious person does not live in a 'cautious mode of self-protection, clinging to our lives desperately at all cost, making an idol of our own physical survival' (10–11).

Although the solution – engagement with God in others or withdrawal from selfhood and material craving – may vary, the provoking experience of emptiness remains the same. And there is probably no marker of this sense of transience greater than adult ageing. From a spiritual perspective, the ageing body becomes the medium through which, chrysalis-like, self-awareness is both achieved and left behind. MacKinlay (2001) associates this transition with the experience of 'going home' as the emptiness behind everyday existence is filled by a closer association with divine reality. According to Laceulle (2013), connecting ageing and spirituality 'transforms these so-called losses that transcend the common language of decline and open up new possibilities for meaning' (2013: 112). Atchley (2012) also highlights spirituality as a core domain targeted for growth by the ageing process and sees this as a progress from doing to being – from activity to an openness to immediate experience. This arises from an increasing experience of loss that leads to a "focus on the inner life, service to others, and deepening connection with the sacred [as] bright spots of growth and development for most elders" (2012: 3). These qualities, he argues, contribute to the perception of wisdom and sagacity as a characteristic of old age.

Strong and weak associations between belief and ageing

In trying to makes sense of these varied reports, it may be possible to identify two versions of the relationship between belief and ageing. These may be thought of as a strong and a weak interpretation. A strong interpretation might go something like

> Spirituality is a natural developmental process that allows older adults to overcome the challenges of a long life. It is the process that achieves meaning

through moving beyond the concerns of the body and the material world and connection to a different form of reality. This reality centres on relationship with supra-natural beings, or transcendental states of being, that are universal in scope and far greater than the self.

A weak interpretation would state that

Spirituality is a coping strategy that allows a certain accommodation to be achieved to suffering through an acceptance of vulnerability and connection to others. It contributes to meaning-making by placing individuals within a broad set of priorities that are greater than those generated by the self alone. Recognising a spiritual dimension to adult ageing allows a reinterpretation of the meaning of ageing as experienced and for adaptation to take place to a state of personal finitude.

Both represent different forms of liminality. The former emphasises an alternative perception based on the divine and a process of increasing awareness of being between material and spiritual realities. The latter places greater emphasis on the social construction of reality and the possibility of introducing an approach to ageing that modifies dominant interpretations of its implications for human limitation and interconnection.

An important factor of spirit as an idiom for ageing is that it does not attempt to ignore or deny important experiences that occur with respect to vulnerability and lack. Indeed, such experiences are included as indicators of transition to a different state of being and a novel set of priorities for adapting to a long life. It offers a specific form of interconnection between self and others and, for believers, God. That other explanatory frameworks, such as productivism and bodily maintenance, leave little space in their internal organisation for the expression of spiritual belief, makes spiritual awareness a persuasive candidate for what is 'hidden' in everyday engagement with the world, something that lies behind the veil of everyday masquerade.

The major religions and ageing

So what do the major religions have to say about the relationship between spirituality and ageing? Perry Anderson (2015), in his review of the work of the historian Dmitri Furman, remarks on the unpopularity of comparative religious study and the difficulties in comparing religions within the western academy. However, as belief systems have a unique perspective on the process of ageing, and while this chapter focusses on what has been said about religious belief systems within gerontological discourse, it also explores the ways in which the major beliefs recognise adult ageing and include it as a factor in spiritual development, at least as they have been picked out by scholars of ageing.

Coleman (2011), reporting on 40 years of the Southampton longitudinal study, notes an increasing diversity of spiritual belief and that many religions are flourishing and bear 'stubborn witness' in the face of both explicit and tacit repression. Three traditions are outlined here, with a special emphasis on their approach to adult ageing and a long life. The Abramic tradition includes, in historical order, Judaism, Christianity and Islam. Another includes Buddhism and Hinduism and a third, Confucianism. Each perceives a liminal relationship between the self and the divine, but the responses that are made to ageing and generational relations include both similarities and stark differences.

The Abramic belief systems teach respect for the old but also point up examples of foolishness as well as wisdom. Each advises on conduct towards the age-other. A long life is seen in the context of a teleological journey with a universal purpose, leading to transcendence. Gordon Harris (2008) points out that 'the Bible', honoured in different forms by each tradition, 'does not directly advise elders about old age or attack ageist stereotypes. It speaks in stories, poetry and character studies' (2008: 12). Each of the Abramic great texts takes the form of oral history that requires the reader to contextualise the ancient context and bracket their own preconceptions. Each makes claims of divine revelation; however, at least in the Christian context, attention to ageing or intergenerational dimensions is rare. Ingram and Loy (2005) note that the Abramic tradition posits a personal self whose continuity through old age, death and beyond is dependent on a creator to whom we remain ultimately responsible. Age is an opportunity to follow in God's ways, be pleasing to him and do good to others.

Wisdom and elderhood are not necessarily related to age, but age is associated with wisdom and can be attained through life experience. And as Rabbi Friedman (2008) points out, older people are assumed to have acquired understanding of God's ways through life experience and are inherently worthy, over and above any capacity to contribute or benefit those younger than themselves. Gordon Harris (2008) says that reference to old age are limited in the New Testament. This may in part be a reflection of the young age at which its founder died in human form and, in part, an emphasis on the inclusive nature of the message and method of induction. He argues that the easiest place to seek specific guidance on adult ageing comes from the Old Testament. Here, later life is often portrayed in interaction with younger generations, either to highlight appropriate and inappropriate forms of conduct, as a guide to the age-other, or with ageing as a reward for a pious life. Age never guarantees wisdom, but intergenerational responses should be protective of dignity, with Noah and his sons giving a postflood example of how not to do it. The relationship between Eli and Samuel exemplifies descent into poor judgement as well as intergenerational partnership. Moses's relationship with first Jethro as a young man and then Joshua as an elder himself and the mentoring relationship of Elijah with Elisha each give a perspective on the proper role of eldership and intergenerational relations. Ecclesiastes offers advice from experience on enjoying the gift of life's fleeting day, mostly concerning positive relationships and accomplishing good, while Job is an example of the eventual rewards of faithfulness.

Mentoring (Gordon Harris, 2008) constitutes the most advanced form of intergenerational relations, including both accountability and commitment to one another. The mentor acts as a model for satisfactory behaviour and values. The understudy is supported, and where possible, success is ensured through empowering an understudy to do the work at hand. The relationship is mutually affirmatory and marked by honest and open communication. It requires judgement and receptiveness plus an emotional bond. Further, a mentor knows when to terminate mentorship and release an understudy into the world without dependency. 'Mentoring advice will not solve pain and losses. Rather, that relationship needs to quietly support a mentored one through pain and grief and leave ultimate restorations and emotional healing to God' (2008: 46).

In his book *Jewish Visions of Ageing*, Friedman (2008) gives advice on the care of others in an intergenerational context, with both a long life and positive conduct towards the age-other being seen as a matter of reward. He points out that: 'while most of the mitzvoth (commandments) in the Torah are mandated without assurance of reward, in a few exceptional cases long life is a promised recompense' (2008: 8). In other words, a long life is a potential consequence of right conduct, especially between generations, and honouring one's parent is the only commandment offering a temporal reward. However, Freidman observes that the Torah is silent about how one must feel about them. One respectfully lends assistance, preserving dignity, but one is not required to love. This, he argues, recognises the complexity of parent-child relationships and the primacy of the middle child-rearing- generation. According to Coleman et al. (2011), Judaism admonishes us not to neglect the old, while Christianity emphasises an ongoing life with God beyond death as a form of witness to the human condition. Thursby (1992) notes that Islam, like Judaism, promotes the family. Authors agree that both conduct towards older adults and a long life, particularly in its bodily manifestation, are valued, principally because they provide an opportunity for spiritual development. Coleman et al. (2011) observe that 'the body is seen primarily as a means for development of the soul. Persons are therefore encouraged to maintain good health, and will be judged accountable for the way they have looked after the blessing of a healthy body and mind' (2011: 147).

Trials associated with an ageing body are a reminder that they are surmountable and temporary and provoke virtues of patience and perseverance. Thursby (1992) notes that the Quran tends to regard the loss of capacities that typically are suffered in old age to be 'only the most obvious evidence of the universal frailty and dependence that is the inevitable condition of all human creatures' with suffering a 'reminder of the overwhelming mercy, justice and power of Allah' (1992: 178). Material existence is limited and as vulnerable as a well-watched orchard in a scorching whirlwind. Awareness of human limitation leads to submission to Allah, who knows the plight of every creature and will reward the faithful on the day of judgement. Moberg (2002) notes that in Islam both health and illness are believed to come from God, and the art of healing is closely linked to worship. 'The body itself is seen as a mere receptacle of the spirit, which alone constitutes the immortal part of human existence' (Iqbal, 1998: 34), and even a difficult old age is regarded by the devout as an opportunity to strive to perform good actions and to remain faithful to God. Family plus the five pillars of faithful observance (testimony, prayer, fasting, charity and pilgrimage) are primarily focussed on the 'state of the heart' rather than the body.

The Hindu and Buddhist traditions are both marked by infinitely long time cycles that allow perfection or dissolution of the self. Ageing appears principally to be seen as an exemplar of why one needs to discipline the body and aim for an ultimate release from suffering. Thursby (1992) points out that just as

> Islam promotes the family. Hinduism reveres the renouncer, but seeks to pro-tect family values by establishing a balance between the claims of worldly responsibility and the call of spiritual pursuits that may require their renuncia-tion. . . . The early and determining orientation of Buddhism was toward the celibate homeless, wandering world renouncer.
>
> (1992: 188)

Hinduism identifies particular stages of lifecourse development, with renounc-ing sages as positive role models in later life (outlined in the following chapter) and has generally positive expectations of people as they become old and, in some interpretations, closer to God. In Thursby's account, the later Upanishads advise a shaking off of the body, with age as evidence of samsara, the endless cycle of life and death from which certain castes seek liberation and use rigorous yogic methods to obtain release. There exists 'an ageless unsullied self within the individual' (184), which experiences reincarnation as if it were a change of clothes. As Ram-Prasad (1995) observes, renunciation is not thought of as rejection of the sort envisaged by western notions of disengagement; rather than a rejection of life, it marks an acceptance of its limited and provisional meaning. A focus on renunciation of the material, unsurprisingly, means that there is a relative lack of concern about ageing, except long life and death as exemplars of earthly suffering or as a product of good karma (Coleman et al., 2011). For Buddhists, the life of Gautama and his path of realisation (and eventual transcendent Buddhahood) occurred largely because he gained insight from four sights: a decrepit old man, a sick man, a dead man and then a renouncing monk. Each exemplified the futility of relying on transient material realities, which are clung to but are ultimately illusory. There is therefore a tendency to focus on the most painful and negative elements of ageing, with an aim to escape from suffering depending on the dissolution of the concept of self (Little & Twiss, 1978). Both Hindu and Buddhist teachings ultimately depend on selflessness or the achievement of an unchanging self through renunciation. Bodily ageing, itself a result of transience, is both problematising and an opportunity, with old age as an example of why one should strive for renunciation.

Confucian teaching differs from the other major religions, in so far as from the outside, it hardly looks like a spiritual pursuit at all. It presents, according to Anderson (2015), as if 'the impersonal order of heaven was alone divine: the seat of truth wisdom and justice, but cold and indifferent to human beings' (2015: 22). If other belief systems have accentuated the future and opportunities for transfor-mation, Confucianism emphasises one's ancestors and the past, hierarchy, author-ity, order, and duty. Thang (2000) notes that this ordering of things, by a celestial bureaucracy and judiciary, offers a conceptually high status for older adults and is often referred to as if it were a preindustrial 'golden age of ageing'. Much of this perception is based on the notion of filial piety: 'benevolence on the part of the senior and willing obedience on the part of the junior' (2000: 196). But it also coexists within a complex web of mutual obligation between generations, so that while a son is expected to take responsibility for his older parents, the parents are expected to build a new family home for him in the family's village. This series of relations has come under some strain in China and elsewhere with younger adult migration to the cities, although grandparents often look after grandchildren while parents are absent for long periods. While the effects on the filial ethic is disputed, change has led to calls for a redefinition of the relationship between the individual and the temporal state (Du & Xie, 2015). According Andersen, however, a strength of Confucian thought, relative to other religions, is that it could coexist with other belief systems as it was basically a social teaching rather than the profession of a single spiritual truth.

If there is a recognised bond between teachings, it can be found in what has been called the Golden Rule. Each of the major traditions accept, in one form or another, that equal consideration of interests should be given to oneself and to others. Thus Jesus (Luke 10:25–28) speaks of the one great commandment, to 'love your neighbour as yourself'. Rabbi Hillel concludes, 'What is hateful to you do not do to thy neighbour'. Both of whom are interpreting Leviticus (19:18). Islamic Hadith (Kitab al-Kafi, vol. 2, p. 146) cite, among others, Mohammad's incident with a Beduin, where he says, 'As you would have people do to you, do to them; and what you dislike to be done to you, don't do to them'. Confucius teaches, 'What you do not want done to yourself, do not do to others' and 'Never impose on others what you would not choose for yourself' (Analects XV.24, tr. Hinton). In the Mahabharata, there are a number of incidences in which we are told, 'Let no man do to another that which would be repugnant/injurious to himself' (Anusasana Parva, Section CXIII, Verse 8), while Buddhism teaches 'Just as I am so are they, just as they are so am I' (Tripitaka, various). Both see selfish desire as a negative influence on dharma and as the cornerstone of ethics.

The Golden Rule takes positive and negative forms: treat others like yourself, and don't do bad things to them. But condenses a universal rule on how interpersonal and therefore intergenerational relations should be conducted. It is this common understanding that addresses vulnerability and lack in a way that is distinctive of the relationship between spirituality and adult ageing.

Concluding comments

A curious quality of the answers given to adult ageing by the major belief systems is that while forms and interpretations and applications may change, the core teachings of each remain strikingly similar. This is perhaps their strength in offering an answer to the 'why' of a long life. The answer is that each, with the possible exception of Confucianism in its non-Taoist form, is aiming at transcendence and preparation for supramaterial identity or dissolution into something universal. Much of the thinking about ageing that one finds in religious teaching appears to address the older adult as an age-other. Even Islam's, Hinduism's and Buddhism's discourses on the body appear to speak as if the body is in some way exterior to the core self, an item that serves lessons and must be overcome. In the Abramic traditions, conduct towards the elder is explained, but much less is said about one's experience of the processes of growing older. So while these teachings speak to the individual, they do so through the medium of a set of universal principles that identify a relationship with the divine or the universe. And while spiritual development takes place over time, ageing is a secondary consequence of this progress, measured against an unchanging ideal. They do not, in other words, focus principally on lifecourse change and adaptation, except as a drift from one side of a liminal transition to another. But because, with the possible exception of Buddhism, each teaching refers to the importance of relationships with others, they do give a template for intergenerational relations within this broader frame. So while there is a tendency to see the old as an age-other, there is also a tendency to value engagement between self and other as a mirror to relations with God. It contains a mixture of 'within' and 'between-age' discourse, which uses the medium of relations with others and the body to achieve personal transformation.

As such, they offer a reply to death and suffering and provide some objectives for adult ageing to negotiate. As one would expect from systems that pretend to universal explanations, each offers a perspective, if differing ones, on ageing as a phenomenon, ageing in relationship and ageing in others. The belief systems summarised here deal with temporal continuity and discontinuity by offering a continuous yet changed identity in which the notion of selfhood is itself subject to radical revision. In terms of discourse on ageing, belief has become the container for thinking and feeling about liminality, of being between states and drawing upon more than one domain to inform change and transformation. In its strong form, it also offers a perspective that converts decline and vulnerability into a launch pad towards a more advanced state of being. The dynamic encapsulated by spiritual discourses on ageing would be that of impending transcendence – how one rises, in other words, above the daily challenges and insights that a long life presents in order to engage with a novel set of purposes. And in many respects, clinging to life projects, such as the maintenance of current lifestyles, midlife priorities and the denial or avoidance of ageing, would be seen as forcefully inhibiting the opening of that process.

The liminal quality of belief presents a continuing negotiation between alternatives. One finds oneself between continuity and change, present and lifetime-centred experience, within- and between-age thinking and universal and diverse forms of experience. Through this process, it offers a narrative on common vulnerability and finitude that is rarely encountered when negotiating other stories of ageing.

References

Anderson, P. (2015). On Dimitri Furman. *London Review of Books*, 37(15), 19–22.
Atchley, R. C. (2009). *Spirituality and aging.* Baltimore, MD: Johns Hopkins University Press.

Atchley, R. C. (2012). Continuity, spiritual growth and coping in later life. In R. E. Mackinley (Ed.), *Aging, spirituality and palliative care* (pp. 19–30). New York, NY: Harworth Press.

Baars, J. (2012). *Aging and the art of living.* Baltimore, MD: Johns Hopkins University Press.

Baltes, P. B., Freund, A. M., & Li, S. (2005). The psychological science of human aging. In M. L. Johnson (Ed.), *The Cambridge handbook of age and ageing* (pp. 47–71). New York, NY: Cambridge University Press.

Baltes, P. B., & Mayer, K. U. (Eds.). (1999). *The Berlin aging study: Aging from 70 to 100, a research project of the Berlin-Brandenburg Academy of Sciences.* Cambridge, England: Cambridge University Press.

Biggs, S. (1999). *The mature imagination: Dynamics of identity in midlife and beyond.* Buckingham, England: Open University Press.

Bion, W. (1962). A theory of thinking. *The International Journal of Psycho-Analysis, 43,* 306–310.

Chatters, L. M., Taylor, R. J., Bullard, K. M., & Jackson, J. S. (2009). Race and ethnic differences in religious involvement: African Americans, Caribbean blacks and non-Hispanic whites. *Ethnic and Racial Studies, 32*(7), 1143–1163.

Cohen, H. L., Thomas, C. L., & Williamson, C. (2008). Religion and spirituality as defined by older adults. *Journal of Gerontological Social Work, 51*(3–4), 284–299.

Cole, T. R. (1992). *The journey of life: A cultural history of aging in America.* New York, NY: Cambridge University Press.

Coleman, P. G. (2011). *Belief and ageing: Spiritual pathways in later life.* Bristol, England: Policy Press.

Coleman, P. G., Begum, A., & Jaleel, S. (2011). Religious difference and age: The growing presence of other faiths. In P. G. Coleman (Ed.), *Belief and ageing: Spiritual pathways in later life* (pp. 139–156). Bristol, England: Policy Press.

Coleman, P. G., Gianelli, M., Mills, M., & Petrov, I. (2011). Religious memory and age: European diversity in historical experience of Christianity. In P. G. Coleman (Ed.), *Belief and ageing: Spiritual pathways in later life* (pp. 113–138). Bristol, England: Policy Press.

Cooper, M. (2017). *Existential therapies.* London, England: Sage.

Dartington, T. (2010). *Managing vulnerability: The underlying dynamics of systems of care.* London, England: Karnac Books.

Davenhill, R. (2008). Psychoanalysis and old age. In R. T. Woods & L. Clare (Eds.), *Handbook of the clinical psychology of ageing* (pp. 473–488). New Jersey, NJ: John Wiley & Sons.

Du, P., & Xie, L. (2015). The use of law to protect and promote age-friendly environment. *Journal of Social Work Practice, 29*(1), 13–21.

Flynn, M. (2015). Personal communication.

Frankl, V. E. (1955). *The doctor and the soul.* New York, NY: Knopf.

Friedman, D. A. (2008). *Jewish visions for aging: A professional guide for fostering wholeness.* Woodstock, VT: Jewish Lights Publishing.

Gordon Harris, J. (2008). *Biblical perspectives on ageing: God and the elderly* (2nd ed.). New York, NY: Harworth Press.

Grenier, A., & Phillison, C. (2014). Rethinking agency in late life. In J. Baars, J. Dohmen, A. Grenier & C. Phillipson (Eds.), *Ageing, meaning and social structure: Connecting critical and humanistic gerontology* (pp. 55–81). Bristol, England: Policy Press.

Harvey, I. S., & Silverman, M. (2007). The role of spirituality in the self-management of chronic illness among older African and Whites. *Journal of Cross-Cultural Gerontology, 22*(2), 205–220.

Hays, R. B., & Hays, J. C. (2003). The Christian practice of growing old: The witness of scripture. In S. Hauerwas, C. Stoneking, K. Meador & D. Cluotier (Eds.), *Growing old in Christ* (pp. 1–19). Grand Rapids, MI: Erdmans.

Holstein, M. B., Waymack, M., & Parks, J. A. (2010). *Ethics, aging, and society: The critical turn*. New York, NY: Springer Publishing Company.

Ingram, P. O., & Loy, D. R. (2005). The self and suffering: A Buddhist-Christian conversation. *Dialog, 44*(1), 98–107.

Iqbal, M. (1998). Islamic medicine: The tradition of spiritual healing. *Science & Spirit, 9*(4), 34–36.

Kaufmann, E. (2010). *Shall the religious inherit the earth: Religion, demography and politics in the 21st century*. London, England: Profile Books.

Kirby, S. E., Coleman, P. G., & Daley, D. (2004). Spirituality and well-being in frail and nonfrail older adults. *The Journals of Gerontology Series B: Psychological Sciences and Social Sciences, 59*(3), 123–129.

Koenig, H. G., McCullough, M. E., & Larson, D. B. (2001). *Handbook of religion and health*. Oxford, England: Oxford University Press.

Laceulle, H. (2013). Self-realisation and ageing: A spiritual perspective. In J. Baars, J. Dohmen, A. Grenier & C. Phillipson (Eds.), *Ageing, meaning and social structure* (pp. 97–118). Bristol, England: Policy Press. DOI:10.1332/policypress/9781447300908.001.0001

Little, D., & Twiss, S. B. (1978). *Comparative religious ethics*. San Francisco, CA: Harper & Row.

MacKinlay, E. (2001). *The spiritual dimension of ageing*. London, England: Jessica Kingsley Publishers.

MacKinlay, E. (2014). *Spirituality of later life: On humor and despair*. Abingdon, UK: Routledge.

Moberg, D. O. (2001). The reality and centrality of spirituality. In D. O. Moberg (Ed.), *Aging and spirituality: Spiritual dimensions of aging theory, research, practice, and policy* (pp. 3–20). Binghamton, NY: Haworth Pastoral Press.

Moberg, D. O. (2002). Assessing and measuring spirituality: Confronting dilemmas of universal and particular evaluative criteria. *Journal of Adult Development, 9*(1), 47–60.

Moody, H. R. (1997). *The five stages of the soul: Charting the spiritual passages that shape our lives*. New York, NY: Doubleday.

Nelson-Becker, H. (2017). *Spirituality, religion and aging*. Chicago, IL: Sage.

Ram-Prasad, C. (1995). A classical Indian philosophical perspective on ageing and the meaning of life. *Ageing and Society, 15*(1), 1–36.

Ridge, D., Williams, I., Anderson, J. E., & Elford, J. (2008). Like a prayer: The role of spirituality and religion for people living with HIV in the UK. *Sociology of Health & Illness, 20*(3), 413–428.

Sadler, E., & Biggs, S. (2006). Exploring the links between spirituality and "successful ageing". *Journal of Social Work Practice, 20*(3), 267–280.

Sadler, E., Biggs, S., & Glaser, K. (2013). Spiritual perspectives of Black Caribbean and White British older adults: Development of a spiritual typology in later life. *Ageing and Society, 33*(3), 511–538.

Sapp, S. (2010). What have religion and spirituality to do with aging? Three approaches. *The Gerontologist, 50*(2), 271–275.

Singer, P. (Ed.). (1991). *A companion to ethics*. Oxford, England: Blackwell.

Taylor, R. J., Chatters, L. M., & Jackson, J. S. (2007). Religious and spiritual involvement among older African Americans, Caribbean Blacks, and non-Hispanic Whites: Findings from the national survey of American life. *Journals of Gerontology: Social Sciences*, *62B*(4), S238–S250.

Thang, L. L. (2000). Aging in the east: Comparative and historical reflections. In T. Cole, R. Kastenbaum & R. Ray (Eds.), *Handbook of the humanities and aging* (2nd ed.) (pp. 183–213). New York, NY: Springer Publishing Company.

Thursby, G. R. (1992). *Islamic, Hindu, and Buddhist conceptions of aging*. New York, NY: Springer Publishing Company.

Tornstam, L. (2005). *Gerotranscendence: A developmental theory of positive aging*. New York, NY: Springer Publishing Company.

Wilkinson, P.J. & Coleman, P.G. (2011). Coping without religious faith: Ageing among British humanists. In P. G. Coleman (Ed.), *Belief and ageing: Spiritual pathways in later life* (pp. 97–112). Bristol: The Policy Press.

Wink, P., & Dillon, M. (2008). Religiousness, spirituality, and psychosocial functioning in late adulthood: Findings from a longitudinal study. *Psychology of Religion and Spirituality*, *S*(1), 102–115.

Zimmer, Z., Jagger, C., Chiu, C. T., Ofstedal, M. B., Rojo, F., & Saito, Y. (2016). Spirituality, religiosity, aging and health in global perspective: A review. *SSM-Population Health*, *2*, 373–381.

6 Lifecourse, gerotranscendence and wisdom

Key themes

- How to negotiate a long life through meaning-making
- From fixed stages to transition points and processes
- Gerotranscendence as a model of age-specific change and positive discontinuity
- Wisdom as a process of self-conscious negotiation of a long life or as a narrative to be resisted
- Both are concerned with within-age thinking
- Aiming for present-centredness within a lifetime context

Time, self and possibility

Running through the discussion in the preceding chapter is a question. It is one that is pertinent to the relationship between belief, spirituality and ageing and concerns the role of time. How does one connect universal belief systems to considerations of lifecourse change, personal development and intergenerational relations? While late modernity is full of uncertainties and insecurities, it also presents all things as being susceptible to revision and renegotiation (Laceulle, 2013), to which notions of a universal cosmic reality, not being easily pinned down and studied, strike a discordant note. Rather than proposing belief as a gateway to an alternate reality, contemporary research has tended to construe it as a social construction, shaped by local cultures and serving an interpretive function as wider social realities themselves change. A shift to consumerism has become characteristic of contemporary identity management, emphasising interchangeability and choice (Bauman, 2004). This also influences patterns of belief. In her Australian study, MacKinlay (2001) found that older individuals who had had a conventional Christian upbringing drew upon Christian and non-Christian sources when constructing spiritual perspectives. In Britain, as in other postindustrial societies, there has been a rise in alternative 'New Age' spiritual movements, often associated with the baby boomer generation (Wink & Dillon, 2008) and a renewed interest in humanism (Wilkinson & Coleman, 2011). These trends have been described as a 'sacralisation of the self' where sacred forces are seen to dwell within the individual and where spirituality includes a range of traditions that individuals draw upon as a matter of choice (Houtman, Aupers & Heelas, 2009). Trends towards the consumption of a pick and mix spirituality have had an increasing if limited appeal. Atchley (2009) identifies this with a search for a personally authentic spirituality unmediated by religious authority. He characterises it as more akin to improvisational theatre than a traditional submission to faith. Under such conditions, it is easier to speak of a spiritual life as a process of seeking answers rather than accepting them from established authority, and as Gilleard (2013) has pointed out, belief and its relationship to ageing has shifted from a preoccupation with medieval purpose to that of modern meaning-making.

If spiritual belief exists as a potential, or as a sense of ill-defined longing or lack, there is debate over whether a spiritual idiom has to be worked at or arises as a natural part of growing older. Atchley (2009) claims that spiritual development can occur both 'naturally and consciously' as one ages, representing the 'higher possibilities of adult development' and that a spiritual narrative can be particularly valuable in understanding lifecourse change. To become an explicit influence on people's lives, however, Moody (1997) argues that

> unlike physical ageing, the spiritual function within a person does not unfold and progress automatically according to a biologically pre-programmed schedule. Our spiritual capacity exists as a possibility only. If it is to unfold . . . it must be intentionally and consistently encouraged over a period of time via struggle, commitment and effort.
>
> (1997: 33)

Spiritual development and the adult lifecourse

While theories of spiritual development assume a direct link between the ageing process and the development of spiritual belief, thinking in this area has tended to follow wider trends in the psychological and social literature and has moved from a consideration of developmental stages towards a closer understanding of the processes involved.

Stages and processes

Of the great religions, Hinduism uniquely proposes a sequence of lifecourse stages, although these are restricted to merchant, warrior and Brahmin castes. The principal objective of the stages would appear to be to reconcile family responsibilities with the spiritual life. In the student stage (Brahmacharya ashrama), unmarried males are tutored by a spiritual master. This is followed by a householder stage, open to both genders, which fosters active responsibility for family and business life (Gridhastha ashrama). Following the birth of grandchildren, a more removed focus on family seniority and decision taking takes priority (Vanaprastha ashrama). In a final stage (Sannyasa ashrama), elders can relinquish familial and social identity and become solitary wanderers, dedicated to spiritual realisation. Each stage highlights specific ethical and social responsibilities, so that spiritual development becomes regulated and predictable. The first three parts of the adult lifecourse gain meaning by being world-oriented, whereas the final stage is devoted to world-transcending devotion (Ram-Prasad, 1995). Ram-Prasad (1995) notes that humans apprehend the spiritual throughout their lives, but it is in old age where it becomes most relevant.

Within the western psychosocial tradition, Peck (1968), working in the late 1960s, drew on Erikson's ego psychology to propose a three-stage model of spiritual development. The first consisted of a tension between ego differentiation and work role preoccupation and in many ways also follows Jung's (1933) thinking on the processes of individuation and the shedding of a social persona in midlife. Peck claimed that this first stage required a 'crucial shift in the value system by which the retiring individual can reappraise and redefine his worth, and can take satisfaction in a broader range of role activities than just the time specific work role' (1968: 91). His concern here was with the purposelessness of retiring men and the discovery of worthwhile roles without a work identity. Peck's model is sequential, in that each stage is seen to follow on from the last. The second stage emphasises bodily transcendence versus body preoccupation. While not giving a chronological age to these stages, he sees it provoked by declining resistance to illness and lessened recuperative powers. Life begins to take the form of 'a decreasing spiral centred around a growing preoccupation with their bodies' (1968: 91), with meaning being achieved by transcending physical discomfort and in spite of disability. The third stage centres on ego transcendence versus ego preoccupation and is shaped by the prospect and fear of personal death. In old age, he argues, you know death is going to come. As MacKinlay (20) points out, 'you wait for it, it does not arrive unexpectedly'. This realisation creates a concern for future generations. What happens after one dies and the dissolution of the ego? This model, particularly in its earlier stages, reflects a world before a disability and anti-ageing movement and a preoccupation with vitamins and the gym. It does, however, raise important questions on the recognition of vulnerability in the self and how this might evolve.

In 1981, Fowler published 'Stages of Faith,' a six-stage model for the development of belief. Sequential stages are proposed across the lifecourse, of which the fifth and six stages relate to mid- and later life. Stage 5, 'conjunctive faith', occurs when the individual in midlife becomes increasingly aware of the interconnection of traditional faith systems and results in a greater openness to humility and interdependence, which Fowler claims is 'rare before 30'. In a final, sixth stage, those who attain it achieve a 'universalising faith,' finding an approach within which a spiritual way of life can be genuinely lived out. However, Fowler points out that only a few people reach this level of performance.

The model has been questioned on a number of accounts. Labouvie-Vief (2000) claims that it is overly cognitive, underplaying emotional and relational bonds, and MacKinlay (2014) criticises its methodology and gender bias, while Sadler, Biggs and Glaser (2013) argue that universalising and interconnective insights do not follow a sequential pattern and might more accurately be described as differing emphases or pathways towards spiritual belief.

An examined life

Moody (1997), following the precepts of psychotherapy and applying them to spiritual workshops, notes that at some point in the lifecourse, one has been able to 'live long enough and made enough mistakes to recognise an unexamined life goes nowhere' (1997: 28). Adult ageing forces us to decide what is important in life and, as McAdams (1993) has pointed out, leads to the integration of coherent life stories. Moody (1997) itemises a list of five steps for spiritual development, including the Call (from the external to the internal world), Search (disengagement from problems of daily living), Struggle (increased commitment to virtuous behaviour especially towards others), Breakthrough (a discovery of new personal faculties) and Return (a desire to give back), which lead to personal and social affirmation via the spirit. Based on interviews with older adults living in the community and in institutional settings, MacKinlay (2001) proposed a number of 'spiritual tasks' in later life. Two core spiritual tasks were (a) finding ultimate meaning in relationship to God or other people in life and (b) finding different ways of responding to meaning-making (through prayer, meditation, art or music). Linked to these core tasks were four 'subtasks' related to (a) transcending loss or disability, (b) seeking 'final meanings' (related to life review), (c) seeking intimacy with God and others, and (d) the search for hope in life. MacKinlay's study points to the interpersonal nature of spirituality in later life, between the individual and God, which positively affects relations with others. 'While there may be a decline in physiological function in ageing, there remains potential for continued growth in the psychosocial and spiritual dimensions' (2001), she says. Sadler et al. (2013) identified four different routes into spirituality arising from their study of black and white community centre members in South London. They found that Black Caribbean older individuals mostly defined spirituality in relation to their belief in a transcendent God, whereas White British older individuals tended to draw upon a wider range of spiritual, religious or secular notions. The routes consisted of four categories of relationship: 'God to self', 'self to God', 'self to universe' and 'self to life'. A 'God to self' relationship involved an increasingly close and personal connection with God as a transcendent and indwelling spirit, directing their everyday actions and conduct with others. The relationship was often provoked by a conversion or calling at an earlier life stage. 'Self to God' narratives described a relationship that had remained stable over time, with continuity of belief having been shaped by a strong religious upbringing. These respondents drew upon their relationship with the divine, through faith in a transcendent and benevolent guiding force in times of need. 'Self to universe' involved a growing awareness of a broader transcendent reality through nature, music or art. Respondents drew upon a broader transcendent reality as they had more time for reflection in later life and did not necessarily connect it to formal religious belief. 'Self to life' respondents reported existential narratives about a finite life span that provoked a need for meaning and purpose in life, but not in relation to a transcendent dimension beyond material existence. Such a route was often provoked by specific life events at work, in education or through the death of a close loved one.

Timing

When we move from process to timing, Moody (1997) maintains that 'Each person has his or her own inner timetable for self-discovery and that the search for meaning cannot be forced. One doesn't make the grass grow, as the Chinese saying goes, by pulling it' (1997: 26).

This sentiment falls in with non-spiritual explanations of change in later life. For example, Baars (2012) refers to kairos, rather than chronological time, as a marker of lifecourse development. Kairos, the notion of the 'right time' to do something, harks to an awareness of rhythms in nature that reflect changing weather conditions, tides of the sea, and seasons, which make it more or less likely that a particular event will be successful or take place at all. An awareness of lifecourse rhythms can be used to 'sensitise human beings to become attentive to nature's subtle and irregular opportunities and limitations' (2012: 226). There are, in other words, good and bad times to do things, and it is important to take advantage of that moment. This is not the same as being 'on time' in Neugarten's (1968) use of the phrase, to denote whether a particular life event, such as having a first child or going to university is in or out of synchrony with current social expectations. Rather, kairos draws attention to the importance of cycles or waves of time that occur naturally but may not be easily recognised under the din of urban, industrial, 24-hour lifestyles. Baars links kairos to the relationship between rhythms of care and vulnerability. Care, he argues 'has its own temporal dynamics . . . both interpersonal parts and the more instrumental part may show unexpected problems or needs and may consequently, change the temporal dimensions of specific situations' (2012: 230).

Both Coleman (2011) and Friedman (2008) note the importance of ritual in marking the passage of time, either as particular life transitions or as a means of giving meaning to cycles of time, such as in the liturgical year. Friedman (2008) has observed that 'religious time' makes a long life less burdensome and performs a connective function to a wider community and to past and future events, through the repetition of important moments of history or from the lives of spiritual figures. Repetition, it is argued, allows a deeper understanding of the significance of events and their relationship to one's own spiritual development.

Continuity, change and midlife spirituality

Narratives of continuity or change in spirituality among older adults has not been examined by more than a handful of studies, and these have tended to report religious practice rather than changes in belief as such. Life events, such as bereavement and onset of illness, have been associated with a decrease in Christian religious observance in a quarter of the Southampton study's respondents (Coleman, Ivani-Chalian & Robinson, 2004). Ingersoll-Dayton, Krause and Morgan's (2002) study of white and African American older adults outlined four trajectories, which they called stable, increasing, decreasing and 'curvilinear', or fluctuating, patterns. A review by Dalby (2006) found only partial evidence of spirituality as a linear developmental process; rather, patterns of both continuity and discontinuity were identified in older people's narratives. A combination of age, changing personal circumstances, gender and cultural context affected patterns of belief. Sadler et al. (2013) found that among white British respondents, changes associated with ill-health, loss and an awareness of a limited future, but also having more time and a slower pace of life, influenced a search for alternative meaning frameworks and coping strategies in later life. Levels of education appeared not to influence these processes.

A number of studies identified midlife as a time when age-related shifts were more likely to happen either as previously important roles are lost and new forms of affirmation need to be discovered (MacKinlay, 2001) or as the building of an inner transition towards growth and higher forms of consciousness. 'Individual appropriation of traditional spiritual resources' acts as a 'sensitising concept' in this regard (Atchley, 2009: 107), assisting in a move from despair to integrity as one journeys from midlife into old age. And as such, these narratives fall in line with a succession of psychosocial observations from Jung (1932/1967), through the psychotherapies (Frankl, 1984; Montero, de Montero & de Vogelfanger, 2012) and into social psychology in which the middle years of life 'probably the decade of the fifties for most persons, represent an important turning point, the restructuring of time and the formulation of new perspectives of self, time and death' (Neugarten, 1968: 141). According to these studies, a change in focus from time since birth till time left to live and from temporal to ultimate meanings reinforces midlife as liminal: the time at which priorities may shift between material and spiritual domains. Tornstam (2005) is not explicit about the relationship between ageing and spirituality but does claim that individuals from midlife onwards experience change, in the self, social and cosmic levels of perspective. The last of these is associated with a new perception of life and death, time and space, a feeling of being connected to past and future generations and with a broader transcendent reality beyond individual life spans.

Gerotranscendence

The theory of gerotranscendence (Tornstam, 1996, 2005) is one position that has gained increasing popularity in the study of ageing, and, unusually for social gerontology, it draws on phenomena very close to spiritual awareness. The relationship between belief and age is largely tacit, although gerotransecendence has become associated with discontinuity in adult experience, universalism and spiritual awakening. It is worth greater consideration in the current context, largely because it posits a specific set of changes in the relationship between later life, sense of self and connection to a wider reality. Tornstam's conclusions draw on a series of ideas from psychotherapy, developmental psychology and social gerontology and for current purposes can be seen to consist of a number of interconnected components.

Tornstam's original studies took place in Denmark and Sweden and included respondents from 52 to 100 years of age (1994). This has been followed up through additional research, with migrant populations (Ahmadi-Lewin, 2001), in nursing studies (Lin et al., 2016), from community and intergenerational perspectives (Buchanan, Lai & Ebel, 2015), the development of mindfulness (Nilsson, Bülow & Kazemi, 2015) and the experience of pilgrimage (Kalavar et al., 2015). A number of characteristics were identified, which Tornstam posits as indicating an age-specific set of issues. These include increased cosmic communion with the universe, a redefinition of time and space, becoming less self-preoccupied and more selective in one's choice of social activity, increased affinity with past generations with an awareness of 'the generational chain rather than the individual link', a decreased interest in material things, and a greater need for solitary meditation in what Tornstam calls 'positive solitude'.

These practices, which can take place from midlife onward, are not, according to Tornstam, a form of social isolation and withdrawal from social activity – Tornstam claims that youth show more feelings of social isolation than do older adults. Rather, they constitute a form of refinement of activity and perspective. In this sense, gerotranscendence can be seen to approximate Baltes and Carstensen's (1996) work on strategies adopted in later life, which include selection, optimisation and compensation, and also Jung's (1933) proposal that in the second half of life, people direct attention to self- development and become increasingly able to see themselves in a wider universal context. Tornstam is emphatic that gerotranscendence is not a defence or coping mechanism and is motivated by continued life satisfaction.

Gerotranscendence relies heavily on the power of discontinuity. Tornstam begins by observing that at every stage of adult life people believe that 'if everything could just continue unchanged as it is now, life would be at its very best. What lies ahead is nothing to look forward to' (2005: 1). In other words, the present time of life is always seen as the best, and this explains a preoccupation with midlife activity continued into later life. However, 'instead of accepting the hidden assumption that good ageing is the same as continuing the midlife pattern indefinitely, we suggest that growing into old age has its very own meaning and character' (2005: 3). This is encapsulated in 'the gerotranscendent individual . . . [who] . . . 'typically experiences a redefinition of the self and of relationships to others and a new understanding of fundamental existential questions' (2005: 3).

Following Erikson, Erikson and Kivnick (1986), gerotranscendence is seen as 'a late stage in a natural process toward maturation and wisdom' 'simply put gerotranscendence is a shift in meta-perspective, from a midlife materialistic and rational vision to a more cosmic and transcendent one, accompanied by an increase in life satisfaction' (1986: 38). It is claimed that 'this process is intrinsic and independent of culture, but modified by specific cultural patterns' (1986 41) and can be accelerated by life crises that provoke a rethinking of life perspectives. Gerotranscendence, therefore, appears to be a self-reinforcing system with its own dynamism, and once it gets going, the pieces fall into place.

As such, gerotranscendence describes a change in direction and a different set of perspectives on life to what had occurred in earlier parts of the lifecourse that is in line with psychodynamic thinking. It suggests that the development of an ageing identity is discontinuous, rather than being marked by a desire for continuity.

Disengagement

The particular form of discontinuity that Tornstam identifies has laid gerotranscendence open to the criticism that it is simply a reworking of processes of disengagement and does not recognise activity as a factor in social inclusion (Jönson & Magnusson, 2001; Adams, 2004). In the 1960s, disengagement theory (Cumming & Henry, 1961) was used to suggest that older adults withdraw from social life, which had a social function, in so far as to make way for rising generations, to allow a period of withdrawal from society and for introspection. Disengagement became a 'social breakdown syndrome' in the hands of writers such as Kuypers and Bengtson (1973) and was characterised as against the interests of older adults. Tornstam and Törnqvist, (2000) have rejected this association, arguing that a misreading of disengagement as forced social exclusion must be contrasted with voluntary forms of 'positive disengagement' arising from gerotranscendence. They created a questionnaire in an attempt to distinguish the two. The danger, Tornstam (1996) argues, is that by pre-judging the value of activity, we force a paradigm on older adults that 'they themselves no longer inhabit' (38).

Erikson et al., in founding an age-stage orientation to adult ageing, maintained that the rightful task of the final and eighth stage of life was 'an integration of the elements in the life that has passed' (1986: 49). Gerotranscendence, by comparison, constitutes a 'more forward and upward direction' (Tornstam, 2005: 48). The theory received a considerable boost when Joan Erikson (co-researcher and spouse of Erik) endorsed it as a ninth stage of development and a revelation to her at the age of 91.

Writers such as Katz (2000) have since satirised activity theory as producing 'busy bodies', which he associates with a North American preoccupation with the moral virtues of activity for its own sake, while Biggs (2004) has drawn attention to the societal substitution of late-life priorities by those of midlife. According to these authors, disengagement has been criticised because it marginalises older people from midlife forms of social inclusion, whereas the core problem may be that we have inadequately explored what the developmental priorities of later life might actually be. Tornstam is nevertheless concerned to distance himself from 'disengagement' which 'implies only a turning inward [while] gerotranscendence implies a new definition of reality' (2005: 47). Tornstam claims that gerotransecendence is related to higher degrees of both social activity and life satisfaction, even though 'the degree of social activity becomes less important in attaining life satisfaction' (2005: 37).

Part of the enduring attraction of the gerotranscendence approach may be that it opens up an alternative to activity and productivism without formulating a social critique of the status quo. Its charm may lie in that it re-enchants a time of life that has been made sterile by external processes of bureaucratisation and measurement (Jönson & Magnusson, 2001). However, its tendency to pick and mix psychodynamic thinking, developmental psychology, critical gerontology and New Age Buddhism has provoked Jonson & Magnusson to call it 're-enchantment with an oriental touch' (2001: 328). Tornstam's choice of a list of exercises, such as 'being a flower' (2005: 197), doesn't help the sceptical reader, especially if one asks why exercises are needed at all for an inherent and natural process. Perhaps its strength lies in that it offers an answer at least to the contents of what a genuinely age-specific set of priorities might be, if not the process.

A closer look at discontinuity and intergenerational relations

The tension between activity and disengagement is an opposition of surprising persistence and possibly marks one of the underlying contradictions of contemporary ageing. And a policy shift emphatically towards productivity raises the debate to one of a political discourse and therefore of wider dispute. In this context, gerotranscendence offers a powerful alternative vision of self-development in later life.

However, Tornstam never really explains why gerotranscendence has failed to receive the material and cultural resources that would allow it to become a legitimate priority for adult ageing. If it is a 'natural progression', why is it suppressed? Suppression implies a process that one would expect would have to be worked at, and the antagonism between hidden and surface elements of identity would have to be explained. If maturation happens anyway, a core question lies in what permits and inhibits its gerotranscendent form.

The theory is also surprisingly silent on the relationship between the gerotranscendent individual and the age-other, except in a rather abstract concern with the chain of generations and a personal rediscovery of oneself in relation to the past. There is little exploration of how gerotranscendence interacts with generational distinctiveness, how, in other words, the transcendent individual perceives and interacts with actual people of a different age group and how they perceive and interact with her or him.

One is also tempted to ask in what sense are these new and inherent contents of later life transcendent? Because they go beyond first half of life conformity, as suggested by Jung, or in the spiritual sense indicated by the major religious traditions? Are they, then, discontinuous without being transcendent? The theory certainly transcends the body, but largely by ignoring it. The ageing body is rarely mentioned except as a signifier of 'the elderly as feeble and weak in order for us to feel sorry for them' (Tornstam, 2005). This sounds like a gaze aimed at the age-other, and not a very flattering one. Little consideration is reserved for bodily ageing as a spur to a new self-understanding, as it is addressed by a spiritual perspective. Neither is it seen as a provoking a greater awareness of vulnerability or lack. As such, the approach falls into the same set of problems as the midlifestylers who are so keenly criticised, in so far as the ageing body is either denied or avoided. A rejection of vulnerability and bodily decline as a 'misery' narrative means that the theory never really joins the gap between a critique of midlifestylism and lack of importance attributed to bodily decline.

The gerotranscendent answer seems to lie in a discontinuous change in late midlife that occurs as a natural event. This consists of a move towards a personal state of mind that is both more individual and seeking connection to wider transcendent themes. As such, it appears to offer a series of answers to the purpose of a long life, at least in terms of self-actualisation. But it stops short of offering a critical analysis of ageing in respect to others, the ageing body and social relations.

Wisdom and ageing

It is impossible to talk about the development of an ageing identity without interrogating the question of wisdom. The connection is both longstanding in many cultures and has been proposed as a desirable end state by developmental theories of adult ageing. Perhaps, most famously, Erikson(1989) has linked wisdom to old age as an alternative to despair. For the lucky ones, 'It is through this last stage that the lifecycle weaves back on itself in its entirety, ultimately integrating maturing forms of hope, will, purpose, competence, fidelity, love, care, into a comprehensive sense of wisdom' (1989: 56).

Age, as we have seen from the previous chapter, can be used as an example of transience, wisdom and foolishness and though there may be differences of emphasis between eastern and western traditions, Jeste and Vahia (2008) maintain that the basic conceptualisation of wisdom does not appear to have changed markedly across cultures and over a period of millennia. Wisdom archetypes can, according to Jungian psychotherapy (Jung, 1931; Middelcoop, 1985; Samuels, Shorter & Plaut, 1986), appear in dreams. Here, the wise elder often acts as a harbinger of change. Wise old men and women can act as mentors and guides but may also be rejected as the bringers of unwelcome news. More recently, the relationship between ageing and wisdom has been suggested as a target for cognitive-behavioural therapies in cases of late-life depression and anxiety (Laidlaw, 2010).

There have been a number of attempts by gerontologists to define wisdom. Birren and Fisher (1990) have defined wisdom as 'the integration of the affective, conative and cognitive aspects of human abilities in response to life's tasks and problems' (1990: 326). This, in the hands of Baltes and his associates, becomes part of a wider means of coping with age-related change. Here, wisdom 'takes gains and losses jointly into account, pays attention to the great heterogeneity in ageing and successful ageing, and views the successful mastery of goals in the face of losses endemic to advanced age as a result of the interplay of selection, compensation and optimisation'. (Baltes & Carstensen, 1996). Baltes and Staudinger (2000), drawing on the Berlin longitudinal study, define this as 'expert knowledge in the fundamental pragmatics of life that permits exceptional insight, judgement and advice about complex and uncertain matters and expertise in the conduct and meaning of life' (2000: 122). When older adults experienced losses, 'interactive minds' and a 'constructive melancholy' helped them better appreciate what they had and how to adapt to a changed situation. Glück and Baltes (2006) found that wise older people are more likely to age successfully. Brugman (2006) has connected wisdom to acknowledging uncertainty and an ability for dialectical thinking, emotional stability and the ability to act under uncertain conditions. Ardelt (2008) identifies three core elements – cognitive ability, transcending and reflection upon one's own opinions, plus empathy and compassion for others.

MacKinlay (2001) identifies a similar theme in her spiritual reading of the wisdom narrative as 'an increased tolerance of uncertainty, a deepening search for meaning in life, including an awareness of the paradoxical and contradictory nature of reality; it involves transcendence of uncertainty and a move from external to internal regulation' (2001: 153). She cites Psalm 90:12: 'Teach us to count our days, that we may gain a wise heart'.

There has been a tradition in this area of asking the wise expert to identify the characteristics of wisdom. Thus, Sternberg (1990) asked 200 professors of art, business, philosophy and physics for their opinions on wisdom. Baltes, Smith and Staudinger (1992) asked clinical psychologists, finding them to be wiser than average and older ones wiser than younger ones. Jeste et al. (2010) undertook a consensus study of '57 wisdom study experts'. Each study has generated lists of attributes and a proneness to cryptic, wisdom-like pronouncements.

Jeste et al. (2010) undertook a Delphi study of characteristics of wisdom and the related concepts of intelligence and spirituality. Forty-nine of the 53 items identified showed significant group differences between the three concepts, with intelligence being more different to wisdom than wisdom was to spirituality. There was general agreement that wisdom was 'uniquely human, a form of advanced cognitive and emotional development that is experience driven and a personal quality, albeit a rare one, which can be learned, increases with age, can be measured and is not likely to be enhanced by taking medication' (2010: 668). Some forms of spirituality, but not religiosity, were related to wisdom. Wisdom was found to differ from intelligence in terms of application of practical knowledge, recognition of common social good and integration of affect and knowledge. So it appears, as Sternberg (2005) opined, 'people may be smart, but not wise' (2005: 11). Wisdom and spirituality overlapped in the areas of emotional components, self-transcendence and sense of well-being. But things can get very 'listy'. The Delphi study identified nine characteristics along cognitive, reflective and affective dimensions as a means of discrimination between their 53 items. The Berlin studies have identified five meta-categories, each with a list of subdescriptors. Sternberg's Yale Studies (1990) identified six categories with subdescriptors.

In a twist on the expert theme, Pillemer (2015) asked 1,200 elders who had signed up to the Cornell Legacy Study what they thought. Under the heading 'Thirty lessons for living. Tried and true advice from the wisest Americans', he collects a surprising conclusion. In the final analysis, the accumulated wisdom is don't worry so much, and once you reach old age, you don't worry about dying.

General consensus is emerging on the relationship between wisdom and ageing. Clayton and Birren (1980) reported, early on, that older respondents were less likely to accept that wisdom comes with age than younger ones. Birren and Fisher (1990) found that wisdom can increase with experience but not necessarily with old age. And Brugman (2000) concludes that in a nutshell, 'one needs to be old and wise to see that wisdom does not come with age' (200: 115). Sternberg (2005) summarises these observations by saying: 'experience does not create wisdom, rather one's ability to profit from and utilise one's experience in a reflective and directed way is what determines how wisdom develops' (2005: 6)

A number of reasons have been suggested as to how the relationship between wisdom and ageing might emerge. Jeste et al. (2010) have pointed to 'a slowing down that makes us more aware of limitation and finitude – more time to do the "philosophic homework" that a long life presents' (2010: 676). So perhaps intelligence is necessary but not sufficient, yet age is necessary but not sufficient as well. People, it appears, do not naturally grow wiser as they age, but the process of ageing does, nonetheless, furnish the raw material for wisdom, such as experience and memories to reflect on and complex, big-picture thinking, including an openness to contradiction and paradox.

In contrast to the preceding discourse, Woodward (2003) has taken a more vibrant approach. She proposes a critique of wisdom in so far as it relies on emotional disengagement and a suppression of anger at inequality and prejudice against women and older women in particular. According to this view, feelings should not be mastered but expressed as 'wise anger'; otherwise, the old are only left with two scripts: a congenial evenness of judgement, which can be portrayed as cantankerousness, irritability and peevishness if it resists established convention. She cites MacDonald's experiences described in 'Look me in the eye' (MacDonald & Rich, 2001) as an example of constructive rage against ageism within the feminist movement. Anger requires confrontation and not detachment, and to suppress anger leads to depression. Those who look to wisdom as a defining feature of the specific contribution of old age, she argues, find themselves caught in acquiescing to the personal thwarting of old age, via ageism, and a simultaneous denial of the feelings associated with it. The energy of a long life cannot then be used creatively. 'Living up to the emotional (or unemotional) standard of wisdom can have the damaging consequence of suppressing the experience of appropriate anger' (Woodward, 2003: 63).

Whether wisdom results in anger or detachment, whether it is open to all or the pursuit of a minority of elders, Erikson et al. (1986) argues that an urge to wisdom is present throughout the lifecourse as a tacit anticipation of the final task of old age. From a humanist standpoint, this may correspond to what Baars (2013) has called 'the art of living'. From a spiritual perspective, it involves capturing the human-divine relationship (MacKinlay, 2001). A common thread might lie in a narrative of fulfilment through a reframing that engages with the past, the present and the future. And whatever lists one has to refer to, this reframing appears to consist of a process of integration and of letting go. Integration may come in many guises. Jung's (1931/1967) process of individuation, a principal task for the second half of life, concerned a rising into consciousness of potential that had previously been suppressed. Moody (1997) sees it in the marrying up of thought and feelings, Erikson et al. (1986) in the coming to terms with past life experiences and McAdams (1993) in the creation of a 'story to live by'. Spiritual discourses have emphasised a process of reframing through letting go, in order to move forward (Fischer, 1985), 'shedding' (Clements, 1990) and 'stripping away' (MacKinlay, 2001). In each case, there is a movement beyond the social and cultural conformities of preceding years and the generation of a novel set of perspectives on oneself, others and wider realities.

Concluding comments

As our understanding of the adult lifecourse has shifted from the progression from fixed stages to an examination of transition points and processes, the connection between spirituality as a guide to liminality and belief as a handbook for transcending the everyday challenges of adult ageing increases. Gerotranscendence and wisdom narratives have a number of common themes in helping us critically apprehend this process. These are also not dissimilar to those associated with psychotherapy in later life (Biggs, 1991). In the case of psychotherapy, the principal goal is to live with the past, in order to move forward. A common feature of each is a concern with the effect of time on identity, and through that, a process of integration and adaptation to the limitations of an ageing body. Spiritual perspectives add to these psychosocial processes by promising hope that transcendence doesn't simply offer a narrative for living a long life but a future beyond it. Hope adds to the contemporary dimension of relationships with others, a universal relationship with the divine. It offers a validation of stepping away from everyday priorities, but its relationship to continuity and discontinuity is ambiguous.

When viewed through the lens of generational intelligence, gerotranscendence feeds into a critical appraisal of wisdom and offers a complementary perspective to interpersonal relations. Gerotranscendence primarily addresses a state of self-development in later life. Both agree with GI in focussing on lifecourse driven changes, the perception of those changes and a consequent re-calibration of psychosocial priorities. However, both are at times more descriptive than explanatory. Neither seriously includes a focus on interconnection between age groups, while later life is seen to have its own meaning and character. There is no attempt, for example to address intergenerational negotiation, other than noting a different perspective from the 'other'. As such, neither are relational in a GI sense, and there is little attempt to explain the processes underlying them, as might be done by linking them to notions of complexity, individuation, separation and return that would be provoked by placing growing older in the context of intergenerational relations. As a consequence, neither approach addresses how these emerging states can be so difficult to express in contemporary ageing and often ageist settings. It is unclear what triggers, facilitates or inhibits preferred states of being. They do not explain their kairos, their timing.

Baltes, Freund and Li (2005) have argued that as we move into a time of life where physical autonomy is more vulnerable, we become increasingly dependent on cultural forms of support. Whereas narratives based on work and productivity rely on continued autonomy, those considered in these two chapters would seem to offer an alternative cultural narrative that outlines a special role for a long life, for which the categories associated with the study of wisdom and spirituality offer the ultimate bucket list. They provide their own answers to our two questions: what is the purpose of a long life, and how can we adapt to changing generational relationships. The field on which they play includes the tension between temporal continuity and discontinuity. And as such they act as a container for liminality, the state of between-ness that can mark the priorities of a long life. The dynamic that is set in motion is our relation to transcendence and how we can adapt to its pull. It is certainly not a discourse that embraces ageing as 'more of the same'. It is a compelling candidate for a maturity that exists beyond a mask of ageing.

References

Adams, K. B. (2004). Changing investment in activities and interests in elders' lives: Theory and measurement. *International Journal of Aging & Human Development, 58*(2), 87–108.

Ahmadi-Lewin, F. (2001). Gerotranscendence and different cultural settings. *Ageing & Society, 21*(4), 395–415.

Ardelt, M. (2008). Wisdom, religiosity, purpose in life, and death attitudes of aging adults. *International Journal of Existential Psychology and Psychotherapy, 2*(1), 138–358.

Atchley, R. C. (2009). *Spirituality and aging*. Baltimore, MD: Johns Hopkins University Press.

Baars, J. (2012). *Aging and the art of living*. Baltimore, MD: Johns Hopkins University Press.

Baars, J. (2013). Critical turns of aging, narrative and time. *International Journal of Ageing and Later Life, 7*(2), 143–165.

Baltes, M. M., & Carstensen, L. L. (1996). The process of successful ageing. *Ageing and Society, 16*(4), 397–422.

Baltes, P. B., Freund, A. M., & Li, S. (2005). The psychological science of human aging. In M. L. Johnson (Ed.), *The Cambridge handbook of age and ageing* (pp. 47–71). New York, NY: Cambridge University Press.

Baltes, P. B., Smith, J., & Staudinger, U. M. (1992). *Wisdom and successful aging*. Lincoln, US: University of Nebraska Press.

Baltes, P. B., & Staudinger, U. M. (2000). Wisdom: A metaheuristic (pragmatic) to orchestrate mind and virtue toward excellence. *American Psychologist, 55*(1), 122–130.

Bauman, Z. (2004). *Wasted lives: Modernity and its outcasts*. London, England: Polity Press.

Biggs, S. (1991). Community care, case management and the psychodynamic perspective. *Journal of Social Work Practice, 5*(1), 71–81.

Biggs, S. (2004). Age, gender, narratives, and masquerades. *Journal of Aging Studies, 18*(1), 45–58.

Birren, J. E., & Fisher, L. M. (1990). The elements of wisdom: Overview and integration. In R. J. Sternberg (Ed.), *Wisdom: Its nature, origins, and development* (pp. 317–332). Cambridge, England: Cambridge University Press.

Brugman, G. M. M. (2000). *Wisdom: Source of narrative coherence & eudaimonia: A lifespan perspective*. Delft, the Netherlands: Eburon.

Brugman, G. M. M. (2006). Wisdom and aging. In J. E. Birren & K. W. Schaie (Eds.), *Handbook of the psychology of aging* (6th ed., pp. 445–476). London, England: Elsevier Academic Press.

Buchanan, J. A., Lai, D., & Ebel, D. (2015). Differences in perception of gerotranscendence behaviors between college students and community-dwelling older adults. *Journal of Aging Studies, 34*, 1–9.

Clayton, V. P., & Birren, J. E. (1980). The development of wisdom across the life span: A reexamination of an ancient topic. *Life-Span Development and Behavior, 3*, 103–135.

Clements, W. M. (1990). Spiritual development in the fourth quarter of life. In J. J. Seeber (Ed.), *Spiritual maturity in the later years* (pp. 55–65). New York, NY: Haworth Press.

Coleman, P. G. (2011). *Belief and ageing: Spiritual pathways in later life*. Bristol, England: Policy Press.

Coleman, P. G., Ivani-Chalian, C., & Robinson, M. (2004). Religious attitudes among British older people: Stability and change in a 20-year longitudinal study. *Ageing and Society*, *24*(2), 167–188.

Cumming, E., & Henry, W. E. (1961). *Growing old, the process of disengagement*. New York, NY: Basic Books.

Dalby, P. (2006). Is there a process of spiritual change or development associated with ageing? A critical review of research. *Aging & Mental Health*, *10*(1), 4–12.

Erikson, E. H. (1989). *The life cycle completed*. New York, NY: W. W. Norton & Company.

Erikson, E. G., Erikson, J. M., & Kivnick, H. Q. (1986). *Vital involvement in old age*. New York, NY: W.W. Norton & Company.

Fischer, K. R. (1985). *Winter grace: Spirituality for the later years*. New York, NY: Paulist Press.

Fowler, J. W. (1981). *Stages of faith the psychology of human development and the quest for meaning*. San Francisco, CA: Harper & Row.

Frankl, V. E. (1984). *Man's search for meaning*. New York, NY: Washington Square.

Friedman, D. A. (2008). *Jewish visions for aging: A professional guide for fostering wholeness*. Woodstock, VT: Jewish Lights Publishing.

Gilleard, C. (2013). Renaissance treatises on "successful ageing". *Ageing and Society*, *33*(2), 189–215.

Glück, J., & Baltes, P. B. (2006). Using the concept of wisdom to enhance the expression of wisdom knowledge: Not the philosopher's dream but differential effects of developmental preparedness. *Psychology and Aging*, *21*(4), 679.

Houtman, D., Aupers, S., & Heelas, P. (2009). Christian religiosity and New Age spirituality: A cross-cultural comparison. *Journal for the Scientific Study of Religion*, *48*(1), 169–179.

Ingersoll-Dayton, B., Krause, N., & Morgan, D. (2002). Religious trajectories and transitions over the life course. *The International Journal of Aging and Human Development*, *55*(1), 51–70.

Jeste, D. V., Ardelt, M., Blazer, D., Kraemer, H. C., Vaillant, G., & Meeks, T. W. (2010). Expert consensus on characteristics of wisdom: A Delphi method study. *The Gerontologist*, *50*(5), 668–680.

Jeste, D. V., & Vahia, I. V. (2008). Comparison of the conceptualization of wisdom in ancient Indian literature with modern views: Focus on the Bhagavad Gita. *Psychiatry: Interpersonal and Biological Processes*, *71*(3), 197–209.

Jönson, H., & Magnusson, J. A. (2001). A new age of old age? Gerotranscendence and the re-enchantment of aging. *Journal of Aging Studies*, *15*(4), 317–331.

Jung, C. G. (1931). *The aims of psychotherapy*. London, England: Routledge.

Jung, C. G. (1931/1967). *Collected works* (Vol. 16). London, England: Routledge.

Jung, C. G. (1932/1967). *Collected works* (Vol. 7). London, England: Routledge.

Jung, C. G. (1933). *Modern man in search of a soul*. London, England: Kegan Paul Trench Trubner, (1955 ed. Harvest Books ISBN 0-15-661206-2).

Kalavar, J. M., Buzinde, C. N., Manuel-Navarrete, D., & Kohli, N. (2015). Gerotranscendence and life satisfaction: Examining age differences at the Maha Kumbha Mela. *Journal of Religion, Spirituality & Aging*, *27*(1), 2–15.

Katz, S. (2000). Busy bodies: Activity, aging and the management of everyday life. *Journal of Aging Studies*, *14*(2), 135–152.

Kuypers, J. A., & Bengtson, V. L. (1973). Social breakdown and competence. *Human Development*, *16*(3), 181–201.

Labouvie-Vief, G. (2000). Affect complexity and views of the transcendent. In P. Young-Eisendrath & M. Miller (Eds.), *The psychology of mature spirituality* (pp. 103–119). London, England: Routledge.

Laceulle, H. (2013). Self-realisation and ageing: A spiritual perspective. In J. Baars, J. Dohmen, A. Grenier & C. Phillipson (Eds.), *Ageing, meaning and social structure*. Bristol, England: Policy Press. DOI:10.1332/policypress/9781447300908.001.0001

Laidlaw, K. (2010). Are attitudes to ageing and wisdom enhancement legitimate targets for CBT for late life depression and anxiety? *Nordic Psychology, 62*(2), 27.

Lin, Y. C., Wang, C. J., & Wang, J. J. (2016). Effects of a gerotranscendence educational program on gerotranscendence recognition, attitude towards aging and behavioral intention towards the elderly in long-term care facilities: A quasi-experimental study. *Nurse Education Today, 36*, 324–329.

Macdonald, B., & Rich, C. (2001). *Look me in the eye: Old women, aging and ageism*. Tampa, FL: Spinsters Ink.

MacKinlay, E. (2001). *The spiritual dimension of ageing*. London, England: Jessica Kingsley Publishers.

MacKinlay, E. (2014). *Spirituality of later life: On humor and despair*. Abingdon, UK: Routledge.

McAdams, D. P. (1993). *The stories we live by: Personal myths and the making of the self*. New York, NY: Guilford Press.

Middelcoop, P. (1985). *The wise old man*. New York, NY: Shambhala.

Montero, G. J., de Montero, A. M. C., & de Vogelfanger, L. S. (2012). *Updating midlife: Psychoanalytic perspectives*. London, England: Karnac Books.

Moody, H. R. (1997). *The five stages of the soul: Charting the spiritual passages that shape our lives*. New York, NY: Doubleday.

Neugarten, B. L. (1968). *Middle age and aging: A reader in social psychology*. Chicago, IL: University of Chicago Press.

Nilsson, H., Bülow, P. H., & Kazemi, A. (2015). Mindful sustainable aging: Advancing a comprehensive approach to the challenges and opportunities of old age. *Europe's Journal of Psychology, 11*(3), 494.

Peck, R. C. (1968). Psychological developments in the second half of life. In B. L. Neugarten (Ed.), *Middle age and aging* (pp. 88–92). Chicago, IL: University of Chicago Press.

Pillemer, K. A. (2015). *30 lessons for living: Tried and true advice from the wisest Americans*. New York, NY: Hudson Street Press.

Ram-Prasad, C. (1995). A classical Indian philosophical perspective on ageing and the meaning of life. *Ageing and Society, 15*(1), 1–36.

Sadler, E., Biggs, S., & Glaser, K. (2013). Spiritual perspectives of Black Caribbean and White British older adults: Development of a spiritual typology in later life. *Ageing and Society, 33*(3), 511–538.

Samuels, A., Shorter, B., & Plaut, F. (1986). *A critical dictionary of jungian analysis*. London, England: Routledge and Kagan-Paul.

Sternberg, R. J. (1990). *Wisdom: Its nature, origins, and development*. Cambridge, England: Cambridge University Press.

Sternberg, R. J. (2005). Older but not wiser? The relationship between age and wisdom. *Ageing International, 30*(1), 5.

Tornstam, L. (1994). Gerotranscendence: A theoretical and empirical exploration. In L. E. Thomas & S. A. Eisenhandler (Eds.), *Aging and the religious dimension* (pp. 202–225). Westport, CT: Greenwood Publishing Group.

Tornstam, L. (1996). Gerotranscendence: A theory about maturing in old age. *Journal of Aging & Identity, 2*(1), 17–36.

Tornstam, L. (2005). *Gerotranscendence: A developmental theory of positive aging*. New York, NY: Springer Publishing Company.

Tornstam, L., & Törnqvist, M. (2000). Nursing staff's interpretations of "gerotranscendental behavior" in the elderly. *Journal of Aging and Identity*, *5*(1), 15–29.

Wilkinson, P. J., & Coleman, P. G. (2011). Coping without religious faith: Ageing among British humanists. In P. G. Coleman (Ed.), *Belief and ageing: Spiritual pathways in later life* (pp. 97–112). Bristol, England: Policy Press.

Wink, P., & Dillon, M. (2008). Religiousness, spirituality, and psychosocial functioning in late adulthood: Findings from a longitudinal study. *Psychology of Religion and Spirituality*, *S*(1), 102–115.

Woodward, K. (2003). Against wisdom: The social politics of anger and aging. *Journal of Aging Studies*, *17*(1), 55–67.

7 The ageing body, the social and the natural

Key themes

- Historical tension between biological and social explanations of ageing
- The interaction of biological, psychological and social aspects of ageing
- Narratives of what is natural and unnatural may be used for political purposes
- A natural life span approach has been used to ration resources to the old
- Premature mortality and functional ageing are critically assessed
- Lifecourse rhythms may form an alternative way of negotiating the experience of ageing

Introduction

A core narrative that needs to be negotiated for a long life concerns mental and physical ageing. Key here is the degree to which the human lifecourse is a social construct or is subject to common developmental phases, which are based in but not necessarily determined by biological processes. The WHO (1998) has pointed out that ageing consists of an interplay of biological, psychological and social processes, which, as Baltes and Carstensen (1999) indicate, become increasingly interdependent as one approaches deep old age. Psychodynamic, psychological and psychosocial approaches to human development each report that the adult lifecourse can be seen as consisting of specific stages or phases, each with its own set of priorities and contradictions to be resolved (Biggs, 1999). In later life, these tensions have been described variously as existential differences between the first and second halves of adult life (Jung, 1932/1967), an increasing awareness of finitude (Jaques, 1965), strains between generativity, integrity and despair (Erikson et al., 1986) and contributing to integrative narrative processes (McAdams, 1993). Whether these phases are inherent to lifecourse development and identify-specific characteristics of later life or principally depend upon social conventions is closely related to debates about what can be considered a natural part of human development and what has been imposed upon it in different historical periods by belief systems and policy priorities. Connecting naturalness and the lifecourse has given rise to heated debate on the degree to which different phases are biologically determined or whether they exist at all outside the social imagination.

There are so many different imperatives, narratives and explanations swarming around bodily ageing. The ageing body is a core factor in how we manage our ageing identities. It is what is first seen when the age-other is looked at and therefore forms a boundary between the internal psychological world of the psyche and the external one of social attitudes. It also acts as a marker of our relationship towards the past and the future. The body, in conjunction with the external environment and our expectations of it, determines the degree of agency we have. If our capacities are in some way impaired, then this influences our ability to effect the world, depending upon the degree to which capabilities are enhanced or restricted by the spaces and places we inhabit. Bodily ageing, both physical and mental, is one of the aspects of a long life that is resisted most of all. It is the thing that both provokes a sense of vulnerability in ourselves and projects disgust and devaluation onto others who exhibit these processes. It becomes part of both Jung's (1931/1967) shadow side of our conscious awareness, 'the thing a person has no wish to be' (1967, 16: 470) and Bollas' (1989) unthought known. It is something we know occurs, but we do our best, culturally speaking, to avoid or deny.

Interpreting biological ageing

Cristofalo et al. (1999) give us the following definition of biological ageing: 'with the passage of time, organisms undergo progressive physiological deterioration that results in increased vulnerability to stress and an increased probability of death' (Cristofalo et al. 1999: 98).

The rate of deterioration in later life may be caused by the cumulative effects of natural selection as genetic adaptation is only transmitted up until the point it is handed on to the next generation, so that changes caused by ageing past that point have little effect (Kirkwood, 2002). At the cellular level, protective and repair mechanisms accumulate damage, and later life evidences a postreproductive unravelling of characteristics that are not passed on and therefore do not get a chance for species adaptation. Evolutionarily speaking, longevity is invisible. However, a number of factors have been applied to explain both positive and negative effects on longevity, including rate of living and metabolic potential, calorific restriction, free radical theory, somatic mutation via background radiation, toxic environments, error-containing proteins, hormonally elevated glucocorticoids and immunological variance (Carnes, 2016).

The way in which the ageing body is perceived and responded to depends upon a series of often tacit assumptions. We are old when we can't do things anymore. We are old when we look old, or more accurately are perceived to look old. The two are related and can be detected in the distinction that has been made between the third and fourth ages. The term 'third age' was coined by Laslett (1987) to refer to the then emerging phenomenon of people who were still fit and healthy following retirement and who entered into a period of 'active ageing'. This was contrasted to a subsequent period of increasing decline and dependency, which became known as the 'fourth age'. The transition from one to the other is, however, more complex than a shift in social roles, depending not only on the interaction between the biological, psychological and social, but also the way that these changes are interpreted. This in turn influences what is seen as a legitimate solution to the problem at hand. If, for example, we see the problems of identity and social engagement as resting on a youthful self, somehow trapped within an increasingly aged and unresponsive body (Featherstone & Hepworth, 1989), the remedies suggested would differ from a view that sees the problem resting in a mature set of priorities that cannot be expressed because of a predominantly ageist environment (Biggs, 1997). One would need to change the body, the other to change social attitudes. One assumes the body is malleable, the other that there are inherent developmental processes at work.

Davis (2004) argues that 'a state of health reflects a potential to adapt actively to new environments' (372). Bodily ageing influences these powers of adaptation. But it also, perhaps most forcefully in human experience, refers to our psychological and social ability to adapt to our own changing bodies. A state of health, in this sense, not only depends upon our understanding of the relationship between what is natural and what is unnatural, what is age or socially determined, what is normal to ageing and what is disease; it also depends upon how we come to understand lifecourse-specific change. If ageing is seen as a natural process, a social construct or as a disease, then the way we adapt culturally to bodily and other forms of ageing will vary accordingly (Post & Binstock, 2004).

Sociology and biology

For historical reasons, sociology has had an ambivalent relationship towards things biological, which originates in the 19th-century attempts of its founders to differentiate it from the natural sciences (Neurath & Cohen, 2012) and holds a continuing fear that biomedicine and neuroscience will come to render social interpretations of ageing redundant (Dumas & Turner, 2015). Understanding social phenomena, it was argued, was dominated by an idealised concept of natural science, taken to be representative of 'objective' knowledge, which had to be challenged for the new social science to emerge. This legacy is present in social gerontology, as evidenced by Baars and Phillipson's (2013) comment, from two leading figures in the development of European thinking on ageing: 'The major problems that ageing people encounter are not the inevitable result of biological senescence, nor of unfortunate decisions, but are constructed through social institutions and through the operation of economic and political forces' (2013: 2).

A tension lies, here, in the degree to which the social construction of adult ageing can itself now explain what were previously thought to be biologically determined phenomena. If an idea is taken for granted as common sense, it is argued, it can take on the qualities of a material truth, and intersubjective consensus about ageing is then treated as if it were an objective fact (Estes, Biggs & Phillipson, 2003). If forms of rationality, such as beliefs about gender, sexual orientation, disability and age 'become naturalised, taken for granted, considered as foundational and required, if they become the terms by which we must live, then our very living depends upon a denial of their historicity, a disavowal of the price we pay' (Butler, in Bell, 2010: 121).

In other words, in order to free ourselves of socially created suppositions about ageing that appear natural, we have to rebel against them. Failing to do so forces us to disavow our own historical and social circumstances. If biological determinism, whilst appearing to be based in objective fact, is itself a social creation, then the degree to which ageing can be thought of as changeable is unnecessarily compromised.

In its first wave, sociological approaches to ageing focussed on the dangers of ignoring structural inequality (Estes, 1979; Phillipson & Walker, 1986). If, it was argued, biological ageing and its application through biomedicine and clinical practice, the translation from 'bench to bedside', dominates, then it's social equivalent, a belief in biological determinism is, through the compelling power of medical science, likely to push aside opportunities for social intervention and change. Estes et al. (2003) have defined biomedicine as "medical techniques that privilege a biological understanding of the human condition and rely on pharmacological and technical innovation for their impetus" (2003: 79). Determinism refers to the view that in the final analysis all things can be reduced to, in this case, their physical bodily causes. The concern behind such an analysis is that social inequalities around gender, race, or in this case age, will be perceived to be 'natural' and political priorities will, if not critically analysed, be presented as if there were no alternative to the status quo. In the case of ageing, sociological thinking has been pivotal in pointing out that poverty and disengagement are not inevitable consequences of growing older but a result of structured dependency (Townsend, 1981), whereby older adults are forcibly excluded from forms of social engagement and power, such as work, and with increasing age are placed in institutional ghettos, in hospitals and residential institutions. An underlying critique lay in unmasking a commonly held assumption that dependency in later life was based on biology and therefore immutable, while in reality it had been brought about by social structural conditions. If the determinants of dependency were social in origin, they could be undone. However, by placing biological and social explanations in opposition to each other, authors of this period came to associate biology with rigidity and sociology with the possibility of diversity and improvement.

A second wave of sociological interest focussed on the body itself and the degree to which bodies were, in fact, malleable. Authors such as Featherstone and Hepworth (1989) became interested in the body as a surface that represented the self. Featherstone noted that 'within consumer culture the body is proclaimed as a vehicle for pleasure. The closer the actual body approximates the idealised images of youth, health, fitness and beauty, the higher its exchange value' (1982: 21).

Here, the notion of a separate 'internal' process of selfhood was questioned. The body became a way in which identity could emerge, provoking a debate in gerontology between those who saw ageing as a process of increasing rigidity that inhibited malleable expression (Hepworth, 2004) and those who thought that ageing was an inevitable process of maturity that could be managed, through engagement with a set of existential questions about meaning and lifecourse change (Biggs, 2004). To what degree, in other words, can we 'choose not to grow old'? In response, Higgs and Gilleard (2014, 2015) re-opened a discussion on the relationship between the third and fourth ages (Laslett, 1987). They argued that a focus on malleability and performance has resulted in a sociology of 'not becoming' old rather than one 'of becoming old differently' (2014: 20). A key issue here has been whether very old people can act on the world and in what way. Higgs and Gilleard have argued that the fourth age is increasingly marked by a void, embodying the most feared and marginalised aspects of adult ageing. This debate has been progressed by Grenier and Phillison (2014) who propose that in deep old age, agency has to be thought of in terms of interdependence between the very old and others, and midlife notions of active independence may no longer apply. In this, they reflect Hazan's (2011) description of deep old age as provoking a sort of autism in communication between younger and older adults to the extent that the experience of old age becomes barely recognisable to others. This shift towards considering the nature of the fourth age highlights the growing influence of biological decline on social gerontological thinking. This is not to say that adult ageing can be reduced to biology, nor that bodies exist in separation from psychosocial relations. The field has not, then, been left to biomedicine, but rather the close interconnection between the biopsychosocial is beginning to be recognised, and new and critical ways of asking questions about agency explored.

The nature of natural and unnatural ageing

In the preceding discussion, the portrayal of biology and the accompanying notion of biological determinism can appear limited and stereotyped. However, arguments about 'nature versus nurture', which dominated debate in the late 20th century, have become exhausted, with the conclusion that: 'everything is a mixture of both and it's all very complicated' (Dennett, 2002: 9).

The debate nevertheless holds within it a number of enduring assumptions about what 'natural ageing' actually consists of, what is natural and, perhaps more interestingly, what is unnatural. Labelling a social phenomenon natural or unnatural moves debates on biology into the domain of sociopolitical discourse. An exclusively natural explanation for adult ageing, in its determinist interpretation, has been the subject of sustained feminist criticism (Gullette, 2017; Pickard, 2014). The notion of unnaturalness has been claimed by writers on ecology (Gerber, 1997) and on the alienating effects of work (Berardi, 2005) as a critical tool to challenge conventional thinking.

In this section, the nature of nature, naturalness and unnaturalness are examined. The tension between what is natural or unnatural and therefore requires clinical intervention shows itself to be an amalgam of physical and social factors. Is, for example, menopause a natural phenomenon or a deviation that requires intervention, or are clinical interventions, such as hormone replacement therapy (HRT), part of a remedy to something that is both natural and perceived to be socially undesirable? The close connection between social forces and the creation of new biomedical phenomena can be seen in the 'discovery' of the male menopause. It is perhaps interesting that just as menopause, like birthing, has been reclaimed as a natural process and as remedies such as HRT have become widely used, a new phenomenon, the male menopause, or andropause (Seigal-Watkins, 2007), has been identified. According to Vainionpää and Topo (2005), the notion of a male menopause has surfaced repeatedly in the 19th and 20th centuries, first provoking remedies based on animal extracts to counteract feelings of reduced social potency and standing, then accompanying the rise of social panic over 'midlife crisis' in the 1960s, when older men experienced increasing intergenerational competition, and most recently with the popularised use of Viagra, a drug originally designed to address cardiovascular problems, which quickly opened new markets responding to sexual recreational needs and dysfunction (Katz & Marshall, 2003). By the beginning of the 21st century, andropause had become a sort of protosyndrome and a new market for pharmaceutical remedies in its own right (Marshall, 2007). Vainionpää and Topo's (2005) history shows how closely the development of social anxieties can be reflected in the development of new products. In countries where payment for intervention depends on private insurance, the status of medical syndrome assumes an economic importance, as it triggers the paid use of new pharmaceuticals. This example evidences a close relationship between socioeconomic interests and the creation of a new phenomenon that has been placed within the domain of medicine. It blurs notions of the natural and unnatural, the biological and the social, suggesting a continuum.

The relative power attributed to nature as an explanatory tool varies from discipline to discipline. Gerber (1997) has noted a longstanding tendency for cultural geographers to ignore nature as an autonomous actor, while environmental historians assign agency to nature. Asdal (2012) argues that the true question lying behind the debate is not what is truly natural but how one can critically examine transformations in nature without reducing culture to nature or nature to culture. These arguments have become increasingly salient as the Anthropocene, a geological epoch shaped by human agency, becomes more evident (Davies, 2016). When everyday understandings of the natural are examined, it becomes clear that usage is both multiple and diverse, referring to facts and values. In Keller's (2008) words, it is 'a quagmire' containing 'slippage between specific natures and generic nature between what is the norm, what is expected' (Keller, 2008: 120). Among the many meanings of 'natural', three stand out. One refers to what is inherent, a potential that is essential to the very constitution of the person, thing or phenomenon in question, without which it would not be what it is. Here, notions of 'a natural athlete' or 'natural teacher' exist in everyday use. A second refers to what is not artificial, not subject to human intervention, as in 'unspoilt countryside', 'natural forest' or the more ambiguous 'natural habitat'. And finally, the third is what is intuitively felt to be right or fair, what can immediately be grasped or reasonably expected, as in 'natural justice'. Such meanings can have subversive as well as conformist implications, as for example in criticising legal systems or in identifying thwarted 'natural potential'. Being natural, by one means or another, connotes authenticity and health. Being unnatural, in so far as it indicates a deviation from a statistical norm or expectation, may also imply a state of unwellness for which remedies may be discovered.

Keller (2008) concludes that uses of natural and unnatural not only provide us with 'a kind of history of the self-evident'; they also fail to do justice to biology's fascination with the kinds of regularity and life rhythms that admit exceptions. Regularities occur most of the time but are primarily based on evolutionary fitness and ecological diversity, which themselves depend on random changes that allow an ability to adapt. Biological conceptions of naturalness, in other words, assume adaptation, flexibility and change, although the change might take time to occur. Naturalness is, then, both inherently patterned and, by degrees, malleable.

Uugla (2010) points out that humans have an ambivalent relationship to nature, which oscillates between romantic devotion and attempts to conquer it. In both cases, it is associated with otherness. Thus concepts such as a natural wilderness 'represents both the untouched and pure, which are worth aiming for, and the untamed and violent, which threaten and destroy human lives' (2010: 79).

The boundary between culture and nature, they argue, not only has emotional resonance, but is also politically regulated. Thus, while the notion of protecting the natural may seem neutral or congenial, it is complex and value laden, involving the designation of boundaries in the relationship between humans and their environment. It is not then something to be searched for or avoided but is a concept to be analysed, its instrumental value assessed and implications evaluated. Because human agency may act as destroyer or rescuer, it requires regulation. Yet hidden within the discourse of environmental regulation lies an assumption that disrupts a boundary between a rigid nature and a malleable social and in some ways reverses them. Take, for example, a priority to protect biodiversity. Biodiversity is assumed to be intrinsic to the natural environment, essential for human survival and welfare, ecosystem resilience and adaptability to changing conditions. Problems are amplified by human stressors, but left to its own devices; nature is both malleable and responsive to altered circumstances.

Taken together, biological science and ecological studies, with their fascination with variety and focus on adaptation, show that a concentration on 'naturalness' by no means implies the rigidity that its social critics imply. They chime well with Davis' (2004) definition of an ability to adapt as a core indicator of health. They also resonate with Baars' (2012) discussion of kairos, the rightness for certain activities in harmony with natural rhythms, such as seasonal planting and harvesting or tacking a sailing boat to the changing winds (see Chapter 7). When focussing on the adult lifecourse, biology and bodily ageing supply certain developmental rhythms, which translate, for reflective beings such as humans, into existential priorities that arise from its own span and logic. Indeed, an awareness of rhythmic as compared to, or in conjunction with, linear change is not strange to social science. Bourdieu (1990), for example, claims that 'practice unfolds in time and . . . its temporal structure, that is its rhythm, tempo, and above all its directionality, is constitutive of its meaning' (1990: 81).

This form of adaptation, based on rhythmic bodily change, also provides the basis for a material understanding of a long life that relies less on the uncertainties of social and economic convention and more on a closer attention to lifecourse development. While a discourse on nature can be used to abjure social impacts on ageing and reinforce social conformity, we should be careful not to eclipse the potentially radical value of naturalness as both inherently adaptive and as a critique of practices that damage and distort the potential of a long life. Focussing on narratives of naturalness may provide both a secure material basis for adult ageing and an antidote to the instrumentalism that often accompanies economic or social imperatives surrounding adult ageing. If there are rhythms to the lifecourse, which allow certain priorities to arise at different times due to its intrinsic nature, then we have a material base from which to resist processes requiring lifecourse uniformity. The natural lifecourse is malleable, not in the sense of being able to choose not to grow old, but in that each phase of development gives rise to inherent existential challenges.

Naturalness, policy and limitation

The years of the welfare state, in Western Europe, referred to by Piketty (2014) as the 'trentes glorieuses', not only contributed to increased longevity but prefigured a form of human flourishing that has been historically unprecedented (see for example Chapter 10 on the value of state support to ageing families). The contributing factors are complex and would also include the development of humanistic psychology in the United States and cultural shifts experienced by post–World War II baby boomers. These and other trends may have contributed to a period allowing inherent qualities of the long life to be made visible, to become more fully formed. Important among these would have been the creating of an adequate pension and the birth of the third age, allowing a period of modest freedom for self-development without the alienating discipline of labour. The 'new feudalism' that Piketty subsequently describes, may in the fullness of time reverse the benefits that were achieved and carried through the lifetimes of that particular cohort. The point here is that a refocusing on narratives of naturalness and rhythm, combined with supporting cultural shifts, may allow the limitations of more linear and uniform narratives of ageing, such as that proposed by extended work discipline, to be perceived more clearly.

Unfortunately the notion of naturalness in connection to the adult lifecourse have rarely been used in the liberational way expressed above. Callaghan (1987, 1995) and Daniels (1988, 2012) have both placed longevity in the context of the costs of an ageing population, arguing that there should be limits to the support to health care for the old. While Daniels (1988) has emphasised the low return on investment that expenditure on older adults supplies, Callaghan (1995) most famously refers to 'the biological rhythm of the lifecycle as a way of providing a biological boundary to medical aspiration' (1995: 23).

Callaghan marshals a number of economic and clinical arguments to support the restriction of what are perceived to be excessive interventions in later life (see Estes et al., 2003).

> It should be the aim of medicine to assist people in successfully passing through the different stages of life . . . there is no good reason why this cycle need be any longer, on average, than now it is in the developed nations: namely, seventy five to eighty two years.
>
> (Callaghan, 1998: 130)

Any future increase 'should be encouraged to come about only as the natural by-product of healthier lifestyles and the consequent reduction of illness in old age' (Callaghan, 1998: 253).

By linking his argument to a chronological age and to public access to health care, reductions on state but not individual spending are sanctioned. The cutoff points for an effective rationing of access appear both arbitrary and with the potential to exacerbate health inequalities. The justification for limiting expenditure, which Callaghan (1987) and Daniels (1988) refer to as a 'natural' or 'normal lifespan' respectively, is then used as a point beyond which public support for health services should not be provided. Support beyond that limit Daniels refers to as 'overbenefitting', although no justification in terms of lifetime contributions are considered. Callaghan, however, places his argument in the context of cultural trends that have refused to accept limits and an intolerance of the inevitability of death. In an argument with uncomfortable parallels to the instrumental 'usefulness' of productivism, Callaghan claimed that 'the average person in good health in the developed countries (and living in a relatively safe environment) already lives long enough to accomplish most reasonable human ends' (1998: 82). And goes on to imagine a Swiftian nightmare where older adults are otherwise condemned to a life of meaningless repetition and eventual atrophy: 'a life perpetually stuck at one stage . . . would soon come to boredom and ennui, with the possibility of significant change arrested and frozen' (1998: 131). In Callaghan's world, then, no development is envisioned for a long life, no existential or spiritual questions are to be grappled with. Rather, a limited if unspecified version of contribution is combined with a disregard for the obligation of others when lifetime need may be at its greatest. As Overall (2003) points out in her philosophical inquiry into longevity, 'Callaghan's notion of "a natural lifespan" is biased against anyone with the inherent capacity to live longer' (2003: 43). 'If an eighty year old woman wants to continue to remain alive simply in order to spend time with her children and grandchildren, read books, watch television and enjoy the sunshine on a warm spring day, I defy apologists such as Callahan to show that such a desire us unreasonable, unjustified, or immoral' (2003: 51).

Callaghan and Daniels were writing principally at a time where political justification was needed for a reduction in support for public services, cost containment, privatisation and entitlement reduction. The forced alliance between antagonistic factors, such as chronology and natural ageing, reflect these instrumental priorities. They occurred as new mechanisms for assessing eligibility to health care became available, although these were sometimes dressed in the clothing of assessing expected quality of life.

An example of what can follow from an uncritical and crudely utilitarian pursuit of what is a 'reasonable' life span can be seen in the debate surrounding quality adjusted life years (QALYs). 'If an extra year of healthy (i.e., good quality) life expectancy is worth one', it was argued, 'then an extra year of unhealthy (i.e., poor quality) life expectancy must be worth less than one' (Williams, 1988: 285). Priority would be given to treatments that would increase the largest number of years of life, which, as younger patients might expect a potentially greater number of years to live than older patients, would include a tacit justification for ineligibility based on age. Given the same treatment, older patients would always score lower than younger patients. As Kenny (2015) observes, the World Bank's *Investing in Health* report (1993) commented favourably on disability adjusted life years as a means of assessing human capital and including an 'age weighting' because 'most societies attach more importance to a year of life lived by a young person or a middle aged adult than to a year of life lived by a child or an elderly person' (World Bank, 1993: 26, 231). QALYs and related measures demonstrate an interdependence between political, economic and biomedical judgements that is not immediately clear until it is placed in the context of the adult lifecourse and tacit age prejudice. And while their use had been questioned by a presidential inquiry in the United States, as early as 1982, and by the United Kingdom's 2001 NHS national service framework, they still have an afterlife in disciplines such as health economics (Comans et al., 2016).

While QALYs may now be less commonly used as a basis for clinical decision making, similar arguments could be raised concerning the emerging popularity of measures of 'premature mortality'. Here, authorities such as the US Centers for Disease Control and Prevention (1986) have noted an age distortion in their use but attribute this to figures 'being dominated by the underlying disease processes of the elderly', suggesting that deaths at younger ages should be weighted more heavily by including years of potential life lost. Premature mortality has become a prominent element of the WHO Action Plan on Non-Communicable Diseases (2013–2020), which includes four disease areas – cardiovascular disease, cancer, chronic lung diseases and diabetes – and has the target to reduce deaths before age 70. Following on from the WHO, the United Nations' Sustainable Development Goal (SDG) Three, aims to reduce premature mortality by one-third by 2030. While 'premature mortality' sounds very reasonable and less economic in motivation and few would want others to die prematurely, age is used as a criterion by which to stop measuring. What happens to persons who slip over into the 70-plus bracket and appear to lose their numeric justification for clinical concern? An exchange in the *Lancet* between Norheim, Jha and Admasu (2015) and Lloyd-Sherlock et al. (2015) takes issue with the former's claim that the SDGs reflect the view that the cutoff is justifiable because 'death is inevitable in old age'. In reply, Lloyd-Sherlock et al. point out that

> a chronologically exclusive pre-mature mortality target sends out a strong signal that years lived beyond a given age, such as 60 years or 70 years, are intrinsically less valuable than those of a younger person. This misconception builds on a flawed tradition in health-care priority setting, which includes an explicit bias against older people (as opposed to people of so-called economically and socially productive ages).
>
> (Lloyd-Sherlock et al. 2015)

In a bid to move away from the chronological assessment of eligibility, and to reconnect with bodily ageing as experienced, the WHO's *World Report on Ageing and Health* (2015) focussed on functional capacity. As Margaret Chan, director-general of the WHO made clear, the report constitutes an attempt to go beyond a disease-based approach: 'Healthy ageing is more than just the absence of disease. For most older people, the maintenance of functional ability has the highest importance. The greatest costs to society are not the expenditures made to foster this functional ability, but the benefits that might be missed if we fail to make the appropriate adaptations and investments' (Chan, in WHO, 2015: viii). Healthy ageing is defined as 'the process of developing and maintaining the functional ability that enables well-being in older age' (2015: 28), and drawing on the language of Sen's (1985) capabilities approach, functional ability

> comprises the health related attributes that enable people to be and to do what they have reason to value. It is made up of the intrinsic capacity of the individual, relevant environmental characteristics and the interactions between the individual and these characteristics. . . . The interaction among these health characteristics will ultimately determine the intrinsic capacity of the individual – that is, the composite of all the physical and mental capacities that an individual can draw on.
>
> (2015: 28–29)

It is but a short and positive step from talking about intrinsic capabilities to the inherent potential that a long life contains, expressed in a facilitative environment. However, a danger lies in the degree to which functional ageing becomes reinterpreted as a yardstick for judging productive potential and thereby a limiting form of social inclusion via productivism (Chapter 3). Within a marketised insurance system, high levels functional capacity can also become a 'risk' to the pension insurer in so far as a healthy individual lives longer and therefore costs more, while medical costs nearly always constellate at the very end of life. This 'risk is then transferred back to the insuree by simultaneously increasing their potential down-payments and reducing the amount they would have each year to live on' (Blake, Cairns & Dowd, 2006). It exhibits one example of the tensions that can exist between intrinsic and instrumental understandings of functional ageing.

Concluding comments

The history of the relationship between social and biological ageing has centred on the relative primacy of the body as a focus of concern. Sociological thinking had initially opposed biological explanations of ageing because of the anxiety that reducing ageing to far stronger discourses associated with medicine would eclipse explanations based on social forms of inequality. Fascination with the body as potentially malleable, while principally based on youth, subsequently raised the question of the limiting nature of bodily ageing and how far it inhibited social expression. Both arguments held to an underlying position that the body and biology were essentially fixed, whilst social aspects of ageing were open to modification through various mechanisms ranging from identity management through to social policy. A more detailed study of biological thinking indicates that narratives associated with nature, naturalness and the unnatural are both more nuanced and allow for degrees of adaptation and rhythm, which can form a stable, yet vulnerable material base for lifecourse analysis. However, naturalness, function and life span have been used with ambivalence in the policy arena. Taken together, these arguments suggest that a focus on inherence, rather than naturalness, may have certain advantages for the study of a long life. Inherent potential gives shape and sense to an adult lifecourse as it evolves and adapts to questions of biological change, existential finitude and challenges of social conformity. Left to its own devices the adult lifecourse may develop through certain intrinsic phases, expressed as psychosocial priorities and emerging from its own internal logic. While social thinking about ageing has focussed on the structural constraints on adult development and the degree to which our bodies can be modified, relatively little energy has been put into what ageing might look like if it were allowed to freely develop under optimal circumstances. Another way of putting this is that in a reaction against a tendency to reduce ageing to physical and mental decline, we have lost contact with the narrative power of what might be inherent and natural in human development and what is, by implication, unnatural. Without this distinction, which allows diversity and is very different to claiming that something is statistically or morally 'normal', the possibility of exploring facilitative social and environmental circumstances is greatly reduced.

We are also left with a contradiction. Bodily ageing is unstable, but not in the right way, not in a way that can be controlled by immediate personal agency because it is 'malleable'. Rather it is imbued both with certainty (growing older and bodily decline) and uncertainty (when, where, how, and the degree to which it can be delayed). Further, our concern with the ageing body is marked by physical and mental continuities and discontinuities: how long can we keep going and what might disrupt our continuing agency? As such, it seeks to contain elements of fear and hope about the future made manifest in our material selves. While the dominant medium is that of health and medicine, its dynamic is largely one of avoidance: how health can be maintained and decline delayed. In the next chapters, we will explore two social phenomena that are extreme reactions to the challenge of a long life. Both are attempts to control our understanding of bodily ageing, for 'us' and for 'them'. One is the development of anti-ageing medicine as an attempt to avoid or deny ageing. The other concerns the social panic and attempts to control fears associated with dementia.

References

Asdal, K. (2012). Contexts in action – and the future of the past in STS. *Science, Technology & Human Values*, *37*(4), 379–403.

Baars, J. (2012). *Aging and the art of living*. Baltimore, MD: Johns Hopkins University Press.

Baars, J., & Phillipson, C. (2013). Connecting meaning with social structure: Theoretical foundations. In J. Baars, J. Dohmen, A. Grenier & C. Phillipson (Eds.), *Ageing, meaning and social structure: Connecting critical and humanistic gerontology* (pp. 11–30). Bristol, England: Policy Press. DOI:10.1332/policypress/9781447300908.001.0001

Baltes, M. M., & Carstensen, L. L. (1999). Social-psychological theories and their applications to aging: From individual to collective. In V. L. Bengtson, J.-E. Ruth & K. W. Schaie (Eds.), *Handbook of theories of aging* (pp. 209–226). New York, NY: Springer Publishing Company.

Bell, V. (2010). New scenes of vulnerability, agency and plurality: An interview with Judith Butler. *Theory, Culture & Society, 27*(1), 130–152.

Berardi, F. (2005). What does the cognitariat mean? Work, desire and depression. *Cultural Studies Review, 11*(2), 57–63.

Biggs, S. (1997). Choosing not to be old? Masks, bodies and identity management in later life. *Ageing and Society, 17*(5), 553–570.

Biggs, S. (1999). *The mature imagination: Dynamics of identity in midlife and beyond.* Buckingham, England: Open University Press.

Biggs, S. (2004). Narratives, masquerades, feminism and gerontology. *Journal of Ageing Studies, 18*(1), 45–58.

Blake, D., Cairns, A. J. G., & Dowd, K. (2006, February). *Living with mortality: Longevity bonds and other mortality-linked securities.* Paper presented to the Faculty of Actuaries and to the Institute of Actuaries, London, United Kingdom.

Bollas, C. (1989). *Forces of destiny: Psychoanalysis and human idiom.* London, England: Free Association Books.

Bourdieu, P. (1990). *The logic of practice.* Stanford, CA: Stanford University Press.

Callaghan, D. (1987). *Setting limits: Medical goals in an aging society.* New York, NY: Simon & Schuster.

Callaghan, D. (1995). Aging and the life cycle: A moral norm? In D. Callaghan, R. H. J. ter Meulen & E. Topinkova (Eds.), *A world growing old: The coming health care challenges* (pp. 20–27). Washington, DC: Georgetown University Press.

Callaghan, D. (1998). *False hopes: Overcoming the obstacles to a sustainable, affordable medicine.* New York, NY: Simon & Schuster.

Carnes, B. A. (2016). *Longevity, biological: The encyclopedia of adulthood and aging.* Chichester, England: Wiley.

Comans, T., Peel, N. M., Hubbard, R. E., Mulligan, A. D., Gray, L., & Scuffham, P. (2016). The increase in healthcare costs associated with frailty in older people discharged to a post-acute transition care program. *Age and Ageing, 45*(2), 317–320.

Cristofalo, V. G., Tresini, M., Francis, M. K., & Volker, C. (1999). Biological theories of senescence. In V. L. Bengston & K. W. Shaie (Eds.), *Handbook of theories of aging* (pp. 98–112). New York, NY: Springer Publishing Company.

Daniels, N. (1988). *Am I my parents' keeper? An essay on justice between the young and the old.* Oxford, England: Oxford University Press.

Daniels, N. (2012). Aging and intergenerational equity. In Global Agenda Council on Aging (Ed.), *Global population ageing: Peril or promise? World economic forum* (pp. 29–34). Retrieved from www3.weforum.org/docs/WEF_GAC_GlobalPopulationAgeing_Report_2012.pdf

Davies, J. (2016). *The birth of the Anthropocene.* Oakland, CA: University of California Press.

Davis, D. H. (2004). Dementia: Sociological and philosophical constructions. *Social Science & Medicine, 58*(2), 369–378.

Dennett, D. Who' afraid of determinism? (2002, December 6). *Times Literary Supplement.*

Dumas, A., & Turner, B. S. (2015). Human longevity, utopia, and solidarity. *The Sociological Quarterly, 56*(1), 1–17.

Erikson, E. H. (1989). *Identity and the life cycle*. New York, NY: International University Press.

Erikson, E. G., Erikson, J. M., & Kivnick, H. Q. (1986). *Vital involvement in old age*. New York, NY: W.W. Norton & Company.

Estes, C. L. (1979). *The aging enterprise*. San Francisco, CA: Jossey-Bass.

Estes, C. L., Biggs, S., & Phillipson, C. (2003). *Social theory, social policy, and ageing: A critical introduction*. Berkshire, England: Open University Press.

Featherstone, M. (1982). The body in consumer culture. *Theory, culture & society, 1*(2), 18–33.

Featherstone, M., & Hepworth, M. (1989). Ageing and old age: Reflections on the postmodern life course. In B. Bytheway, T. Keil, P. Allatt & A. Bryman (Eds.), *Becoming and being old: Sociological approaches to later life* (pp. 143–157). London, England: Sage.

Gerber, J. (1997). Beyond dualism – the social construction of nature and the natural and social constructions of human beings. *Progress in Human Geography, 21*(1), 1–17.

Grenier, A., & Phillison, C. (2014). Rethinking agency in late life. In J. Baars, J. Dohmen, A. Grenier & C. Phillippson (Eds.), *Ageing, meaning and social structure: Connecting critical and humanistic gerontology* (pp. 55–81). Bristol, England: Policy Press.

Gullette, M. M. (2017). *Ending ageism or how not to shoot old people*. New Brunswick, NJ: Rutgers University Press.

Hazan, H. (2011). Gerontological autism: Terms of accountability in the cultural study of the category of the fourth age. *Ageing and Society, 31*(7), 1125–1140.

Hepworth, M. (2004). Embodied agency, decline and the mask of ageing. In E. Tulle (Ed.), *Old age and agency* (pp. 125–136). New York, NY: Nova.

Higgs, P., & Gilleard, C. (2014). Frailty, abjection and the "othering" of the fourth age. *Health Sociology Review, 23*(1), 10–19.

Higgs, P., & Gilleard, C. (2015). *Rethinking old age: Theorising the fourth age*. Basingstoke, England: Palgrave Macmillan.

Jaques, E. (1965). Death and the mid-life crisis. *The International Journal of Psycho-Analysis, 46*, 502.

Jung, C. G. (1931/1967). *Collected works* (Vol. 16). London, England: Routledge.

Jung, C. G. (1932/1967). *Collected works* (Vol. 7). London, England: Routledge.

Katz, S., & Marshall, B. (2003). New sex for old: Lifestyle, consumerism, and the ethics of aging well. *Journal of Aging Studies, 17*(1), 3–16.

Keller, E. F. (2008). Nature and the natural. *BioSocieties, 3*(2), 117–124.

Kenny, K. E. (2015). The biopolitics of global health: Life and death in neoliberal time. *Journal of Sociology, 51*(1), 9–27.

Kirkwood, T. B. (2002). Evolution of ageing. *Mechanisms of Ageing and Development, 123*(7), 737–745.

Laslett, P. (1987). The emergence of the third age. *Ageing & Society, 7*(2), 133–160.

Lloyd-Sherlock, P., Ebrahim, S., McKee, M., Prince, M., & nine signatories. (2015, May 30). A premature mortality target for the SDG for health is ageist. *The Lancet, 385*, 2147–2148.

Marshall, B. (2007). Climacteric redux? Remedicalising the male menopause. *Men & Masculinities, 9*, 509–529.

McAdams, D. (1993). *The stories we live by*. New York, NY: Morrow.

Neurath, M., & Cohen, R. S. (Eds.). (2012). *Empiricism and sociology* (Vol. 1). New York: Springer Science & Business Media.

Norheim, O. F., Jha, P., & Admasu, K. (2015). Avoiding 40% of the premature deaths in each country, 2010–30: Review of national mortality trends to help quantify the UN sustainable development goal for health. *The Lancet, 2*(385), 239–252.

Overall, C. (2003). *Aging, death & human longevity.* Berkeley, LA: California University Press.

Phillipson, C., & Walker, A. (1986). *Ageing and social policy.* Aldershot, England: Gower.

Pickard, S. (2014). Biology as destiny? Rethinking embodiment in "deep" old age. *Ageing and Society, 34*(8), 1279–1291.

Piketty, T. (2014). *Capital in the twenty-first century: The dynamics of inequality, wealth, and growth.* Cambridge, MA: The Belknap Press of Harvard University Press.

Post, S. G., & Binstock, R. H. (Eds.). (2004). *The fountain of youth: Cultural, scientific, and ethical perspectives on a biomedical goal.* London, England: Oxford University Press.

Seigal-Watkins, E. (2007). The medicalisation of the male menopause in America. *Social History of Medicine, 20*(2), 369–388.

Sen, A. (1985). *Commodities and capabilities.* New York, NY: Elsevier.

Townsend, P. (1981). The structured dependency of the elderly: A creation of social policy in the twentieth century. *Ageing and Society, 1*(1), 5–28.

United States Centers for Disease Control and Prevention. (1986). Premature mortality in the United States. Retrieved from www.cdc.gov/mmwr/preview/mmwrhtml/00001773. htm

Uugla, Y. (2010). What is this thing called "natural"? The nature-culture divide in climate change and biodiversity. *Journal of Political Ecology, 17,* 79–91.

Vainionpää, K., & Topo, P. (2005). The making of an ageing disease: The male menopause in Finnish medical literature. *Ageing & Society, 25*(6), 815–840.

Williams, A. (1988). The importance of quality of life in policy decisions. In S. Walker & R. Rosser (Eds.), *Quality of life: Assessment and application.* (pp. 165–172). Boston, MA: MIT Press.

World Bank. (1993). *World development report 1993: Investing in health.* Oxford: Oxford University Press.

World Health Organization. (1998). *Growing older: Staying well: Ageing and physical activity in everyday life.* Prepared by Heikkinen R. L. Geneva, Switzerland: Author.

World Health Organization. (2013). Action plan on non communicable diseases (2013–2020). Retrieved from www.who.int/nmh/events/ncd_action_plan/en/

World Health Organization. (2015). World report on ageing and health. Retrieved from http://apps.who.int/iris/bitstream/10665/186463/1/9789240694811_eng.pdf?ua=1

8 Anti-ageing

Key themes

- Prolongevism as an extension of the life span beyond existing natural limits
- Anti-ageing claims to extend preventative techniques to enhance ageing
- Debate exists between proponents of anti-ageing medicine and bioscientists as to its effectiveness
- The possibility of slowing ageing can create a longevity dividend
- Cultural drift toward the privatisation of responsibility for health and ageing
- Potential increases in social inequality have been hypothesised
- A within-ageing debate about continuity aims at avoiding finitude

Can we delay or even abolish ageing?

Perhaps the most extreme direction that the debate on the body and ageing has taken has been in the area of anti-ageing, the claim that science can delay and perhaps even abolish ageing entirely. This is part of a wider discussion on prolongevism: the extension of the lifecourse beyond existing chronological limits.

Debates on anti-ageing connect a number of narratives on the quality and purpose of a long life. These include the release of natural human potential in later life, consumerism aimed at avoiding the signs of ageing, the adaptability of biology and identity, and the co-option of preventative medical discourse to extend and enhance human performance. It is part of a popular cultural trend for a 'liberation of ageing from old age' (Gilleard & Higgs, 2005), cultural trends that have been summed up as 'everyone wants a long life – no one wants to grow old' (Biggs, 1999). The Pew Research Center's (2013) 'Living to 120 and beyond' survey of American views on ageing, medical advances and radical life extension found that 63% of adults believed prolongevism is 'generally good, and that extending life beyond 120 years would be a 'good thing for society,' and 38% would take such treatment themselves. However, 66% believed that only the wealthy would actually receive it. Interest has been such that in the same year Google created Calico, the California Life Company, to extend human longevity.

Were the claims for prolongevism to be true, they would radically shift debates on longevity with significant consequences for the functioning and purpose of clinical intervention upon one's sense of self, relations between generations and social policy, not least in terms of the balance between personal and collective planning.

Science, prolongevism and aspirational realities

Extraordinary claims are being made about the ability to increase longevity and perhaps abolish decline and postpone death almost inevitably. While each of these claims is slightly different, they have been grouped under the general rubric of 'prolongevism' (Overall, 2003). At the beginning of the 21st century, these claims have appeared under the banners of bioscience and of anti-ageing medicine, labels that distinguish two opposing camps where the territories of scientific rigour and clinical effectiveness have been fiercely disputed. The popular attraction of the prolongevist debate may lie in the ultimate denial of the great unthought-known, that now, we may not only be tempted never to think about personal finitude; we may no longer even have to. The proposal of increased healthy longevity and even the extension of a decline-free lifecourse beyond current limits is not exactly an example 'commonsense reality', where shared cultural assumptions are taken as facts for everyday purposes. Rather, it enters into a social space of future possibility, an 'aspirational reality' (Moulaert, personal communication, 2015), which while not yet and perhaps not ever real, engages with popular desires in such a way as to influence future planning and infinite procrastination. If these aspirational futures come to pass, their impacts on the lifecourse, equality of access and intergenerational relations would push us into areas that are as yet uncharted. If they are false, yet nevertheless aspirationally 'real', then both individuals and societies could fail to address pressing problems of physical and mental competence associated with deep old age. Finally, if they are foreseeable, yet not acknowledged, they could generate a huge missed opportunity.

The case for extending life beyond existing natural life spans has been advanced by the philosopher Overall (2003). In contrast to Callaghan's (1998) pondering on the pointlessness of a long life, Overall (2003) claims that 'most human beings do not have the chance during their lives to realise their potential' and that in order to lead 'full human lives, in the sense of being long and in the sense of being rich with opportunities' (2003: 183–184), they require longer to live. She advances a human potential argument, whereby

> prolongevism advocates the extension of human life in at least a minimum of health, comfort, and well being . . . to employ social and medical means to lengthen the lives of human beings whose capacities for emotion, perception, thought, and action are to at least some degree intact.

> (2003: 191)

Arguing that life is the precondition for all else that we might want, she maintains that a prolonged life would provide the advantages of acquiring additional and varied experiences; continuing to enjoy and repeat forms of intellectual, aesthetic, or recreational activities; pursuing open-ended projects involving artistic, scientific or intellectual inquiry; and holding prospects for self-transformation. Although why an existing life span should not be re-shaped to allow for such possibilities is not addressed, she maintains that an extended life should be a matter of personal choice.

Anti-ageing medicine

Anti-ageing medicine (AAM) presents challenges not only to mainstream understandings of the role of medicine but also to our notions of the natural and unnatural (Post & Binstock, 2004). The debate surrounding it should be distinguished from everyday attempts to sell us 'anti-ageing' cosmetics, although in terms of social attitudes, they are quite closely related. Cosmetic attempts to hide or delay ageing are primarily concerned with the manipulation of appearance. They are concerned with responding to social pressure, and as Gullette (2004) has puckishly remarked, in a society that valued ageing, we might be tattooing ourselves with wrinkles instead. Many of these cosmetic approaches float on an underlying set assumptions that arise from AAM, which itself aims to redefine our perspective on ageing, longevity and the role of clinical practice. Anti-ageing medicine goes beyond the arguments of the longevity dividend (see Chapter 4), that public health interventions and social environments might be used to delay the onset of dependency and decline, to claim that we can potentially cure ourselves of the process of ageing itself. In the words of De Grey et al. (2002), an advocate of the anti-ageing approach, 'it is patently not yet science fact . . . but it has crossed the boundary into science forseeable'. Interviewed by Weiner (2010), De Grey believes that many people alive today will go on to live for 1,000 years or more. De Grey is editor in chief of the journal *Rejuvenation Research*, which regularly monitors developments in this field.

The anti-ageing vision

Much of the activity around anti-ageing medicine has centred around the American Academy of Anti-Aging Medicine (A4M), registered as a non-profit organisation in the United States. The academy trains and certifies physicians, with Klatz, the co-founder of the academy in 1993, claiming a membership of approximately 26,000 practitioners by 2011 and members in 110 countries. The A4M offers a mix of advice ranging from conventional diet and exercise through to the sale of anti-ageing products. However, these activities have not been recognised by mainstream bodies, such as the American Medical Association, and claims and counterclaims of scientific respectability have led to legal and professional dispute. According to Klatz and Goldman (2004: 1), 'Anti aging medicine is founded on the application of advanced scientific and medical technologies for the early detection, prevention, treatment, and reversal of age-related dysfunction, disorders and diseases'.

In 2008, the A4M's house journal, *Anti-Aging Medical News*, maintained (Patti, 2008) that

> whether you call it 'anti-aging' or 'regenerative' or 'restorative' or 'functional'; this is no myth. The last two decades in medicine proves that applied correctly this new genre of medicine results in greater than a 90% resolution of symptoms such as fatigue, insomnia, decreased libido, weight gain, anxiety, depression, muscle and joint pains and decreased mental function. It also results in greater than an 80% improvement of disease states such as fibromyalgia, rheumatoid arthritis, chronic fatigue syndrome, gastric reflux, IBS, high cholesterol, high blood pressure, PMS, PCOS, infertility and in teenagers, ADD, anxiety and sleep disorders.
>
> (2008: 116)

By 2011, greater emphasis was being placed on lifestyle changes but with a continued association with A4M products:

> Antiaging medicine is a lifestyle; there are no 'magic bullet' medicines. As we age, a series of biological changes take place in the body. Anti Aging physicians seek to understand these age-related declines in order to enable a better grasp of the potential for contemporary medical discoveries and applications of biomedical technology to retard or reverse the otherwise inevitable process of senescence.
>
> (Klatz, 2011: 1)

Enthusiasts for anti-ageing medicine, such as Stuckelberger (2008), have built on the WHO's functional capacity model (Kalache & Kickbusch, 1997) but take it to a new level. The original model showed that the speed of age-related decline could be significantly reduced by changes in the environment so that entering a 'disability threshold' would be delayed, forming a basis for the age-friendly cities initiative. Stukelberger argued that anti-ageing pushes beyond what she re-names the 'better ageing' of the WHO, to create a third trajectory, which plateaus as 'peak performance' and includes both human enhancement and a prolonged life. Thus, she uses conventional discourse on preventative medicine to distinguish between 'usual ageing' involving decline and maintenance, 'better ageing' of healthier ageing practices leading to prevention and finally peaking in 'life extension'. Unfortunately, at the time of writing, there was no recognised means of measuring biological age as compared to chronological age, for which functional age is a proxy (Moreira, 2015). In Stukelberger's model, however, anti-ageing medicine becomes portrayed as part of a continuum, originating in mainstream practice and ending in a sustained and higher level of performance. The model sits well and provides conceptual support for Klatz's (2015) position that anti-ageing medicine consists of

> a healthcare model promoting innovative science and research to prolong the healthy life span in humans. As such, anti-aging medicine is based on principles of sound and responsible medical care that are consistent with those

applied in other preventive health specialties . . . Undeniably, anti-aging medicine is achieving demonstrable and objective results that beneficially impact the degenerative diseases of aging.

(2015: 1)

In his article, Klatz extends the horizons of A4M to include the growing market of robotics; artificial organs, such as pancreas and retinas; artificial blood; wearable health monitors and neural interfaces.

As such, anti-ageing discourse supplies a heady picture of anti-establishment, yet clinically sound innovation, now based on a model connected to, yet travelling beyond, mainstream thinking. It is supported by moral claims that to do nothing risks the deaths of 100,000 people a day (Vijg & De Grey, 2014), that it is only a matter of time before it comes fully into being and that time depends upon investment.

The association with mainstream medicine, however, cloaks a clash of ideologies that present a very different view of what medicine should be about. Where conventional medicine specialises in therapy, to get people back to normal functioning, A4M focusses on the extension of current capacities to create enhanced performance. Instead of ethical non-maleficence, to do no harm, anti-ageing promotes beneficence. Instead of assuming that it is normal to age, it invites an equally strong cultural assumption: that it is normal to seek progress. Further, if Mykytyn (2008) is right, it draws upon our humane sentiments in so far as 'liberation of the pain of ageing is a more natural or human pursuit than is the biological decline of ageing naturally'. In many ways, it reflects a split between the assumptive realities of public and commercial service, of collective or individual good, of two sides of the western cultural project. Anti-ageing presents not only a different set of protoclinical activities; it presents a different way of seeing.

The relation to bioscience

A criticism of the anti-ageing approach is that it adopts the language of medical science, preventive medicine and 'New Age' lifestyles to obtain a legitimacy that it does not deserve. As early as 2002, leading figures in the study of biogerontology Olshansky, Hayflick and Carnes came together to express their concerns

> that when proponents of anti-aging medicine claim that the fountain of youth has already been discovered, it negatively affects the credibility of serious scientific research efforts on aging. Because aging is the greatest risk factor for the leading causes of death and other age-related pathologies, more attention must be paid to the study of these universally underlying processes.

> Successful efforts to slow the rate of ageing would certainly have dramatic health benefits for the population, by far exceeding the anticipated changes in health and length of life that would result from the complete elimination of heart disease, cancer, stroke, and other age-associated diseases and disorders'
> (Olshansky, Hayflick & Carnes, 2002: B295).

In an interview for *Science* (2013a), Olshansky repeats the key elements of an argument for new scientific research initiatives:

> The only way to achieve healthy life extension is to slow the aging process, because that influences in a positive way all diseases and disorders simultaneously. It's much more economical to extend healthy life by slowing the aging process than by attacking specific diseases. So, the goal is to increase the length of healthy life. If we continue with the current disease-specific approach, we may prolong life with frailty and disease.
>
> (Olshansky, 2013a: 1)

A position statement by key researchers in this area, including Rowe, co-author of the seminal *Successful Ageing* (Rowe & Kahn, 1998, 2015) argue that 'heart disease, cancer, stroke, and Alzheimer's disease, cluster within individuals as they reach older ages' and ask 'whether we can decelerate the process by which the cluster of conditions described above arises, making people healthier at older ages and even lowering spending on health care. . . . Simply put, can we age more slowly thereby delaying the onset and progression of all fatal and disabling diseases simultaneously?' (Goldman et al., 2013:7, 14). Kaeberlein, Rabinovitch and Martin (2015) argue in *Science* for a move away from biomedical research focussed on individual disease processes to studying relationships between ageing and disease. Longitudinal centenarian studies are being carried out in at least eight countries and have identified factors as diverse as high levels of vitamins A, D and E, certain enzymes and inheriting a hyperactive version of telomerase, which prevents cells from deteriorating. Results can be grouped into 27 genetic signatures, subgroups of centenarians who have that genetic profile in common (Sebastiani et al., 2013). The New England Centenarian Study, begun in 1994, has, for example, identified "281 genetic markers that are 61% accurate in predicting who is 100 years old, 73% accurate in predicting who is 102 years old or older and 85% accurate in predicting who is 105 years old or older" (2015: 1). Nikolich-Žugich et al. (2016) have called for bioscientists and health professionals to form a common alliance to promote a 'healthspan' approach. In an interview in *Nature Medicine* with leading biogerontologists, increased healthspan is explained as efforts to extend the period of healthy life by slowing the biological process so that one year of clock time is matched by less than one year of biological time (Hayden, 2014). The infirmities of old age can, it is argued, be compressed into a short period at the end of life, which currently relies on public health initiatives, including better diet, exercise and disease prevention. Tackling individual disease processes can be frustrating to physicians because at the compressed stage the curing of one disease can simply lead to a patient dying of another. Ageing is, however, described as

> messy; different species age at different rates, different groups within species age at different rates and different organs within individuals age at different

rates. Indeed, nobody knows what 'dying from natural causes' means . . . aging is likely to be a highly polygenic trait.

(2014: 12)

These researchers admit that at the time of writing, study has principally been undertaken with mice and roundworms, plus studies of centenarians and the tie to life extension in the average human population has yet to be developed. It assumes that there is an underlying process that is universal to all age-related diseases that can be identified. However, it is a long step from age being a risk factor correlated with a series of chronic diseases and it being a causal mechanism with a common physical source.

Nevertheless, the project of 'slowing ageing' has been used to connect the social agenda of a longevity dividend to bioscience and genetic research. At one level, it poses the question: how can we learn from populations that actually appear to age slowly or at least live into deep old age to increase longevity for all? And on another, it asks how we can scale up advances made with invertebrates and small mammals into humans. However, it does not ask the perhaps obvious question of how tackling health inequalities via risk associated with living and working conditions, plus access to health care, education and public works (OECD, 2016) might achieve similar collective results.

A tension here lies in whether ageing can be treated as a uniform substrate of a number of factors, or whether it is a coming together of a series of diverse processes and complex interactions, which, whilst arriving at the same end point, have little else in common. That age is a common risk factor in a number of diseases and degenerative processes may not mean that they all hail from one underlying and curable mechanism. There may be no magic bullet, although our understanding of biological ageing may be substantially enhanced. Further, hitching the wagon of a longevity dividend to the pulling power of biomedicine may significantly underplay the value of public health, social and environmental initiatives to provide extra years of healthy life. And, of course, extra years of healthy life and the proposed dividends of lower health care spending and greater productive engagement can take place without prolongevism at all by improving the life circumstances of those living a naturally occurring life span.

A common trajectory

In spite of their antagonisms, the claims of both prolongevist camps, the anti-ageing enthusiasts and the bioscientists have certain areas of common ground. And these implications would have considerable import for future medicine and public policy.

Both appear to agree with the view that, in De Grey et al.'s (2002) words, we are dealing with 'science foreseeable'. They agree that the outcome could be a 'one-stop cure' and consists of the view that in future one form of treatment can be used to address what are currently a collection of deficits and diseases associated with growing older. Both concur that the ultimate goal is, by different degrees, to 'cure' us of ageing, either by prolonging the lives of those whose capacities, as Overall

(2003) said, 'are to at least some degree intact' or by Olshansky's (2013b) 'slowing ageing' to such a degree that, as Vijg and De Grey (2014) maintain, it will abolish suffering and lead to multicentenarial lifecourses. Both wings of the prolongevist paradigm approve of preventive approaches that start in midlife or even earlier in the human lifecourse. Thus, Olshansky et al. (2006) indicate that 'with this effort, we believe it will be possible to intervene in aging among the baby boom cohorts, and all generations after them would enjoy the health and economic benefits of delayed aging'. They were writing in 2006 when the oldest boomers would be in their late fifties. Patti (2008) asks, '*Is anti-aging for you?* Take yourself for a moment to age 50. You have the rest and the best of your life in front of you. How do you want to live these years?' And Stuckelberger (2008) points out that 'in contrast to geriatric medicine, anti-ageing medicine is not primarily targeting the oldest old or centenarians, but rather a wide range of ages among the healthy population starting at an ever earlier age' (2008: 79).

The main difference seems to be that while the former requires scientific funding to pursue the quest, the other maintains that their products are already (almost) there. Whichever is true, the target market can be pushed back to increasingly younger ages.

Commercialisation of longevity

Some authors have suggested that the above is most likely a territorial dispute for legitimacy and financial backing (Fishman, Binstock & Lambrix, 2008). It is not difficult to draw parallels here with the claims of prolongevism and what Estes (1979) has called the 'ageing enterprise', the attempts of professional groups and other interests to define questions about growing old to their own advantage. The enterprise here connects two meanings of the term – first as a new endeavour marking out as yet unexplored territory and second as a new market opportunity. If one accepts Ehrenreich and Ehrenreich's (1971) analysis that "the primary function of the health care system is not the delivery of services but, rather, the pursuit of profits, with secondary functions of research and education" (1971: 166), then it is not difficult to see how easily attempts to locate a fountain of youth or elixir of life (Post & Binstock, 2004) fit the aspirationally real in the everyday, scientific and commercial worlds. As indicated above, the market extends beyond the old to include midlifers and even earlier cohorts. In terms of purchasing preventive and life extension products, the earlier you start, the better. Estes and associates (2001) maintain that this constitutes a commodification of ageing as a source of new market opportunities, while also disguising social remedies and social inequalities associated with age. A process that occurs largely because the logic of the market is one in which individual purchasers and suppliers meet in a neutral marketplace to effect an exchange and then return to their own private activities. Katz and Gish (2015), for example, identify the growth of cosmetic rejuvenation and medical spa clinics, which Marshall (2015) identifies as part of wider trends towards increasingly individualistic and consumption-based anchors for identity in contemporary societies. The growth of new business opportunities around ageing and anti-ageing in particular is undeniable. However, according to *Nature Medicine* (Hayden, 2014), the launch of new companies has produced 'a series of false dawns and side effects' (2014: 20). Scott and DeFrancesco (2015) claim that since 1995, nine new-wave companies were thriving (four of whom had begun in the year of publication), five were classified as 'walking dead' and eight as 'extinct'. Petersen and Krisjansen (2015) observe that the bioeconomy exploits promises of anti-ageing but does not deliver, concluding that 'those who invest heavily in the "bio-economy" on the premise of future wealth and wellbeing would be well advised to hedge their bets'(2015: 42).

Social, personal and political consequences

The prolongevist debate has added a new dimension to the promise of a long life. According to Dumas and Turner (2007), 'because World Bank economists have seen the ageing and low fertility of the developed world as significant threats to continuing global economic growth and social stability, there is considerable interest in the commercial possibilities of stem cell research as a feature of regenerative medicine' (2007: 7).

How to fit productivist and prolongevist narratives together has therefore become a considerable concern. It is one that goes to the heart of the prolongevist dilemma if it is not to be simply seen as adding to the 'problem' of an ageing population by creating ever longer lives. A number of attempts have been made to forsee a solution, with varying degrees of policy weight.

Klatz (2009) has proposed a 12-point plan to improve health care by 2050. The plan includes a number of public schemes to provide support for healthy living, such as subsidised gym membership and one-stop diagnostic and monitoring of prolongevist lifestyles. Included would be the recognition of anti-ageing medicine as a prescribed remedy for ageing processes and support for consumer information and business initiatives in this area. Klatz's argument maintains that

> The global financial meltdown of 2008 has led to an accelerated adjustment of economic reality for billions of people worldwide. Indeed, technologies such as automation and robotics will become more utilized and thus displace the need to have humans in 8 out of 10 of every service and support job. As a result, millions of people will not be needed in the workforce, thus giving rise to The Leisure Class. . . . It will become necessary for nations to establish a Social Contract for The Leisure Class, which subsidizes free education, entertainment, housing, food, and healthcare for this segment of the population and provides incentives for them to still be positive contributors to society at-large. For, The Leisure Class gives rise to a new crop of artists, poets, and creative minds to fuel the next Renaissance Age.
>
> (2009: 6)

It is not clear from this analysis how these newly unemployed yet long-lived populations will access the income necessary to participate in society and deliver the cultural benefits that are proposed. New anti-ageing technologies are seen as part of a technological solution to a dilemma of surplus human capacity, which, drawing on the wider tradition of the anti-ageing movement (Vincent, 2008; Mykytyn, 2008) creates new libertarian and utopian possibilities. Anti-ageing is thereby seen to provide the motor for cultural rebirth. However, the vision is short on how the newly dispossessed achieve access to prolongevist solutions, nor, given longstanding commitment to private enterprise within the anti-ageist movement (Cardona, 2008), how these newly leisured potential consumers access these new markets, other than via public subsidy. That would exacerbate the problem of too many economically dependent older adults, unless a radical redistribution of wealth is achieved within society.

Overall (2003) has, independently and possibly unintentionally, proposed a solution to Klatz's dilemma. She argues for 'affirmative prolongevism', whereby the most disadvantaged would be the first to benefit from anti-ageing approaches. As many humans do not, during their current expected life spans, have the opportunities to realise their potential, the argument goes, those who have experienced particular disadvantage should be offered more time to experience life's goods. She appeals to a sense of social justice to support this proposal in so far as every human being should be able to approach the maximum human life span while compressing morbidity and that each should enjoy fair and equal opportunities to access new technologies of this type. Reasons why younger generations might agree to support prolongevism would be that their 'own parents, grandparents, friends and co-workers' will benefit and 'because one will oneself some day likely be elderly' (2003: 194–195).

However, Overall's policy is not wholly unconditional. As noted earlier, her proposals include those with existing physical and mental capacity, to which is added a 'responsibility to look after oneself' (2003: 196). By implication, its relevance to elders already in the fourth age of dependency would be limited. Men are also excluded from her affirmative regime in so far as, while living shorter lives than women, and therefore suitable candidates for prolongevist approaches, they are not considered to be disadvantaged. The fiscal support and social engineering required to put Overall's proposal into effect would be considerable and tend to be eclipsed by its partial, yet absolutist, appeal to social justice. The willingness of other generational groups to support this form of social change would be an important indicator of success.

To address the burden narrative associated with longevity, both Klatz and Overall would still need to explain how increasing life expectancy alone can create wider benefits to humanity. Their proposals face a considerable policy barrier in so far as they promote extending longevity even further, when the main problem, repeatedly identified by an economic assessment of population ageing, is that fiscally speaking, people are living too long already. This problem could be summarised in the seemingly naïve, yet potent question 'Why are we spending so much on longevity research when we don't know how we will pay for the older people who already exist?'

The notion that ageing societies are actually economically beneficial to all generations has been take up by a number of high-profile gerontologists (Olshansky et al., 2006; Butler et al., 2008; Bloom, Canning & Fink, 2010; Beard et al., 2012). In answer to the question 'Why are societies in the developed world spending so much on longevity research and simultaneously worrying about the burden of increasing numbers of pensioners?' it is proposed that both contribute to increased economic prosperity. Rather than generating a 'longevity gap', the gap between how long people live and the finances they have available to support themselves, bioscience and productivity go hand in hand in so far as they generate a 'longevity dividend'. The new relation between life extension and productivity is put most clearly below:

> In addition to the obvious health benefits, enormous economic benefits would accrue from the extension of healthy life. By extending the time in the lifespan when higher levels of physical and mental capacity are expressed, people would remain in the labor force longer, personal income and savings would increase, age-entitlement programs would face less pressure from shifting demographics, and there is reason to believe that national economies would flourish. The science of aging has the potential to produce what we refer to as a 'Longevity Dividend' in the form of social, economic, and health bonuses both for individuals and entire populations – a dividend that would begin with generations currently alive and continue for all that follow.
>
> (Olshansky et al., 2006: 2)

Butler et al. (2008) give a number of reasons why ageing societies increase wealth, productivity and new markets. These include observations that most discretionary funds are accumulated by populations 50 and above, especially 50 to 65; most private intergenerational transfers go from old to young, not from young to old; healthy individuals have accumulated more savings and investments by their old age than individuals beset by illness; healthy older persons are more apt to remain productively engaged in society in their old age through continuing work or voluntary activity; healthy older persons require fewer health services and they promote growth of 'mature' industries in health care and pharmaceuticals, financial services, insurance and the built environment.

The policy implications of the 'longevity dividend' play well against a backdrop of cultural trends such as the desire to extend midlife lifestyles for as long as possible (Hepworth, 2004). The combination of biomedicine and productive ageing coming together to solve the problem of ageing societies is extremely tempting and taps deeply embedded cultural myths. One might almost say it promises the elixir of life and the alchemist's stone in one. It sounds too good to be true. And it is here that we need to return to the experience of the ageing self and of age-others in the form of generational relationships.

A problem with combining work and longevity as solutions to population ageing has been identified by Cardona (2008), who concentrates on the relationship between public and collective responsibilities for the risks associated with old age and what are seen as becoming private responsibilities. As Phillipson

(1998) has argued, the welfare state bracketed out certain risks from the experience of ageing, through the loss of work (pensions) and the loss of bodily function (health care). This bracketing was achieved through a public acceptance of collective responsibility for members of society who were judged to be vulnerable and dependent. Cardona maintains that anti-ageing effectively replaces welfarism with a form of privatised self-surveillance and responsibility. 'Anti-ageing ideologies', she argues, 'address the three main anxieties and risks individuals face in later life: loss of functionality and sexual appeal, the need to remain employable and to avoid poverty, and a fear of becoming a burden on the family' (2008: 480).

This new source of protection from the negative effects of ageing generates a particular kind of 'care of the self', obsessed with the passing of time and the physical body, which is seen as radical because it challenges the narrative of decline and decay. It gives birth to a 'responsible self', which combines a fear of ageing and dependency with a tendency to self-monitor so that achieving and maintaining health becomes a consequence of personal choices. Because this new solution pays less attention to the effects of physical, social and economic environments, which determine an individual's life chances, it effectively privatises risk and absolves the state from responsibility for its ageing citizens. Further, the notion of social legitimacy is redefined so that 'irresponsible' actions can provoke social exclusion through ageing bodies that have not been well tended. Cardona (2008) argues we are all now cast as private entrepreneurs, even to the extent of avoiding ageing.

A second problem exists in that in addition to underplaying existing health inequalities, the prolongevist project creates what Dumas and Turner (2015) have called 'techno-economic transformations . . . creating new sites of vulnerability that are masked by medical utopias of good health and "living forever"'. In this context, it is unlikely that such technologies will be able to overcome inequalities in distribution and may well exacerbate various forms of injustice' (2015: 1).

While prolongevism creates new markets for 'keeping people alive longer', these authors assume that access exists in a climate of economic scarcity. This, they suggest, will produce forms of 'moral queueing' whereby Cardona's successful, healthy and productive entrepreneurs take precedence, and, over time, the possibility of a 'two species society': those who age normally and those who extend their life spans. Taken together, these arguments predict a world in which persons are blamed for their lack of health and social and political institutions are absolved of their responsibility, leaving the resource rich, who can afford this investment in life extension, as beneficiaries.

Concluding comments

In terms of the purpose of a long life, life extension talks in terms of more years rather than of distinctiveness or value. And while it responds to the anxieties of midlife, it acts on the premise of avoiding or denying ageing processes rather than looking to them as a guide to appropriate action. As such, it confuses longevity with continued youth and misses out on the advantages or value of a long life as a life lived for a long time with its own and different existential priorities. Further, it replaces these priorities with those of a particular form of social inclusion that subsists on the priorities of an earlier part of the adult lifecourse. Whilst seemingly promising to abolish ageing, it plays into a dynamic of social ageism based on present-centred thinking and negative othering of the ageing process and those who exhibit it. Unsurprisingly, this debate ignores the intergenerational implications of longevity as enhancement, in the headlong scrabble to live for as long as possible. The negotiation of intergenerationally sustainable solutions would be a key missing element to be addressed, which leads it to exhibit a 'within-age' approach to social issues, except where these extend to preventative new markets.

A core part of its 'new paradigm' claim appears to be that we are addressing the extension of healthy ageing and need be less concerned with the amelioration of the processes of decline and decay. In addition to the proposal that the human lifecourse can be increased, it is also claimed that longevity can be addressed as a singularity and that the key is contained in early intervention to arrest ageing itself rather than particular disease elements.

It is not the concern here to pass judgement on the effectiveness of claims made, rather to note that the prolongevist debate taps into fantasies and folk myths about the denial of adult ageing as if a continuum flowed from established clinical and medical approaches to a new and underresourced solution to the 'problem of old age'. These aspirational realities challenge notions of 'the natural', arguing in their strong case that age can be effectively abolished and, in a weaker version, slowed down. For health sciences and clinical practice, they propose a new way of looking and responding, re-alignment of the morality of medicine and an assumption that access and inequality are problems easily solved. It is predominantly a within-age approach because of its twin targets of ever longer lives and the abolition of ageing as a meaningful category. As such, it eschews positive discontinuity whilst declining to say what the purpose of a prolonged life might be beyond work or the continued consumption of anti-ageing solutions. It is in this sense that it is present- rather than lifetime-centred. The cultural adaptation to a long life appears to be to further extend it without due consideration of the challenges it might provoke to intergenerational and other forms of inequality.

References

Beard, J., Biggs, S., Bloom, D., Fried, L., Hogan, P., Kalache, R., & Olshansky, J. (2012). *Global population ageing: Peril or promise?* Geneva, Switzerland: World Economic Forum.

Biggs, S. (1999). *The mature imagination: Dynamics of identity in midlife and beyond.* Buckingham, England: Open University Press.

Bloom, D. E., Canning, D., & Fink, G. (2010). Implications of population ageing for economic growth. *Oxford Review of Economic Policy, 26*(4), 583–612.

Butler, R. N., Miller, R. A., Perry, D., Carnes, B. A., Williams, T. F., Cassel, C., & Martin, G. M. (2008). New model of health promotion and disease prevention for the 21st century. *British Medical Journal, 337*, 149–150.

Callaghan, D. (1998). *False hopes: Overcoming the obstacles to a sustainable, affordable medicine*. New York, NY: Simon & Schuster.

Cardona, B. (2008). "Healthy ageing" policies and anti-ageing ideologies and practices: On the exercise of responsibility. *Medicine, Health Care and Philosophy, 11*(4), 475–483.

de Grey, A. D., Ames, B. N., Andersen, J. K., Bartke, A., Campisi, J., Heward, C. B., . . . Stock, G. (2002). Time to talk SENS: Critiquing the immutability of human aging. *Annals of the New York Academy of Sciences, 959*, 452–462.

Dumas, A., & Turner, B. S. (2007). The life-extension project: A sociological critique. *Health Sociology Review, 16*(1), 5–17.

Dumas, A., & Turner, B. S. (2015). Human longevity, utopia, and solidarity. *The Sociological Quarterly, 56*(1), 1–17.

Ehrenreich, B., & Ehrenreich, J. (1971). *The American health empire: Power, profits, and politics*. New York, NY: Vintage/Random House.

Estes, C. L. (1979). *The aging enterprise*. San Francisco, CA: Jossey-Bass.

Estes, C. L., & Associates. (2001). *Social policy and aging: A critical perspective*. London, England: Sage.

Fishman, J. R., Binstock, R. H., & Lambrix, M. A. (2008). Anti-aging science: The emergence, maintenance, and enhancement of a discipline. *Journal of Aging Studies, 22*(4), 295–303.

Gilleard, C., & Higgs, P. (2005). *Contexts of ageing: Class, cohort and community*. Cambridge, UK: Polity Press.

Goldman, D. P., Cutler, D., Rowe, J. W., Michaud, P. C., Sullivan, J., Peneva, D., & Olshansky, S. J. (2013). Substantial health and economic returns from delayed aging may warrant a new focus for medical research. *Health Affairs, 32*(10), 1698–1705.

Gullette, M. M. (2004). *Aged by culture*. Chicago, IL: University of Chicago Press.

Hayden, E. C. (2014). Regulators asked to consider innovative trial design. *Nature Medicine, 20*, 12.

Hepworth, M. (2004). Embodied agency, decline and the mask of ageing. In E. Tulle (Ed.), *Old age and agency* (pp. 125–136). New York, NY: Nova.

Kaeberlein, M., Rabinovitch, P. S., & Martin, G. M. (2015). Healthy aging: The ultimate preventative medicine. *Science, 350*(6265), 1191–1193.

Kalache, A., & Kickbusch, I. (1997). A global strategy for healthy ageing. *World Health, 50*, 2–5.

Katz, S., & Gish, J. (2015). Aging in the biosocial order: Repairing time and cosmetic rejuvenation in a medical spa clinic. *The Sociological Quarterly, 56*, 40–61.

Klatz, R. (2009). *The A4M twelve-point actionable healthcare plan: A blueprint for a low cost, high yield wellness model of healthcare*. The American Academy of Anti-Aging Medicine, A4M. Retrieved May 1, 2017, from www.worldhealth.net

Klatz, R. (2011). "Age-Less" medicine. Interview with Ronald Klatz, MD, DO. Retrieved September 11, 2015, from http://ndnr.com/anti-aging/age-less-medicine-interview-with-ronald-klatz-md-do/

Klatz, R. (2015). Introduction to the science of anti-aging medicine: A state-of-the-specialty review. *Jacobs Journal of Gerontology, 1*(1), 1–7.

Klatz, R., & Goldman, R. (Eds.). (2004). *Anti-aging therapeutics*. Chicago, IL: A4M Conference.

Marshall, B. L. (2015). Anti-ageing and identities. In J. Twigg & W. Martin (Eds.), *Routledge handbook of cultural gerontology* (pp. 210–216). Abingdon, UK: Routledge.

Moreira, T. (2015). Unsettling standards: The biological age controversy. *The Sociological Quarterly*, *56*(1), 18–39.

Moulaert, T. (2015). Personal communication.

Mykytyn, C. E. (2008). Medicalizing the optimal: Anti-aging medicine and the quandary of intervention. *Journal of Aging Studies*, *22*, 313–321.

Nikolich-Žugich, J., Goldman, D. P., Cohen, P. R., Cortese, D., Fontana, L., Kennedy, B. K., . . . Richardson, A. (2016). Preparing for an aging world: Engaging biogerontologists, geriatricians, and the society. *The Journals of Gerontology Series A: Biological Sciences and Medical Sciences*, *71*(4), 435–444.

OECD. (2016). Heath inequalities. Retrieved January 12, 2016, from www.oecd.org/health/inequalities-in-health.htm

Olshansky, S. J. (2013a, October 8). The secret of antiaging is worth looking for: Interview with J. Olshansky. *Science*. Retrieved January 12, 2016, from www.sciencemag.org/news/2013/10/secret-antiaging-worth-looking

Olshansky, S. J. (2013b). Delayed aging: The next big thing? Interview with Jay Olshansky. *Senior Planet*. Retrieved January 12, 2016, from http://seniorplanet.org/delayed-aging-the-next-big-thing/

Olshansky, S. J., Hayflick, L., & Carnes, B. A. (2002). Position statement on human aging. *The Journals of Gerontology Series A: Biological Sciences and Medical Sciences*, *57*(8), B292–B297.

Olshansky, S. J., Perry, D., Miller, R. A., & Butler, R. N. (2006). In pursuit of the longevity dividend. *The Scientist*, *20*(3), 28–36.

Overall, C. (2003). *Aging, death & human longevity*. Berkeley, LA: California University Press.

Patti, S. (2008, Winter). Anti-aging: Myth or reality? *Anti-Aging Medical News*, 116–120.

Petersen, A., & Krisjansen, I. (2015). Assembling "the bioeconomy": Exploiting the power of the promissory life sciences. *Journal of Sociology*, *51*(1), 28–46.

Pew Research Center. (2013). Living to 120 and beyond living to 120 and beyond: Americans' views on aging, medical advances, and radical life extension. Retrieved January 12, 2016, from www.pewforum.org/2013/08/06/living-to-120-and-beyond-americans-views-on-aging-medical-advances-and-radical-life-extension/

Phillipson, C. (1998). *Reconstructing old age: New agendas in social theory and practice*. London, England: Sage.

Post, S. G., & Binstock, R. H. (Eds.). (2004). *The fountain of youth: Cultural, scientific, and ethical perspectives on a biomedical goal*. London, England: Oxford University Press.

Rowe, J. W., & Kahn, R. L. (1998). *Successful aging*. New York, NY: Pantheon Books.

Rowe, J. W., & Kahn, R. L. (2015). Successful aging 2.0: Conceptual expansions for the 21st century. *Journals of Gerontology: Series B, Psychological Sciences and Social Sciences*, *70*(4), 593–596.

Scott, C., & DeFrancesco, L. (2015). Selling long life. *Nature Biotechnology*, *33*, 31–40.

Sebastiani, P., Bae, H., Sun, F. X., Andersen, S. L., Daw, E. W., Malovini, A., . . . Perls, T. T. (2013). Meta-analysis of genetic variants associated with human exceptional longevity. *Aging*, *5*(9), 653–661.

Stuckelberger, A. (2008). *Anti-ageing medicine: Myths and chances*. Zurich, Switzerland: Vdf Hochschulverlag.

Vijg, J., & De Grey, A. D. (2014). Innovating aging: Promises and pitfalls on the road to life extension. *Gerontology, 60*(4), 373–380.

Vincent, J. A. (2008). The cultural construction old age as a biological phenomenon: Science and anti-ageing technologies. *Journal of Aging Studies, 22*(4), 331–339.

Weiner, J. (2010). *Long for this world: The strange science of immortality*. New York, NY: Ecco.

9   Dementia

Key themes

- Dementia as an instance of negative othering
- Evidence of strong popular cultural images
- The growth of a disease narrative
- Tensions between emotional labour and person-centred approaches
- Dementia and social inequalities
- Rights-based initiatives by people living with dementia

From prolongevism to dementia

In previous chapters, we saw how prolongivists have argued for a bright future in extending life for as long as possible but also how the lifecourse has become increasingly commodified raising questions of what is considered natural and unnatural, healthy and unhealthy. The other side of bodily and mental ageing, as something that lets us down and makes our personal and social identity increasingly vulnerable, is most forcefully felt when considering dementia. Both narratives connect to a form of aspirational reality, one positive, the other negative. Both also connect to the hope generated by developments in bioscience, which are both promised, and at the time of writing, remote. In public debate, dementia is most often conceived as a threat to government finances, as a source of moral panic, and as symbolic of ageing in general. It constitutes the journey from existing as a person to becoming an uncooperative and empty body requiring management. Dementia has come to be the fearsome doppelganger of prolongevist promises and harbinger of Swiftian purposelessness.

According to the World Alzheimer's Report (Prince et al., 2015), there are an estimated 46.8 million people worldwide living with dementia in 2015. This number is predicted to reach 74.7 million in 2030 and 131.5 million in 2050. Fifty-eight percent of people with dementia live in low- and middle-income countries, but by 2050, this will rise to 68% in China, India, and their South Asian and Western Pacific neighbours. The US Centers for Disease Control and Prevention (2016) cites prevalence data for specific causes of dementia, indicating that up to 5.3 million Americans have Alzheimer's disease. Starting at age 65, the risk of developing the disease doubles every five years. By age 85 years and older, between 25% and 50% of people will exhibit signs of Alzheimer's disease (Hebert et al., 2013). A meta-analysis (Prince et al., 2014) found global prevalence of dementia from all causes to be between 5% and 7% of adults age 60 plus. Comparing two (Matthews et al., 2013) prevalence surveys of adults age 65 and over almost two decades apart (1989 and 2008), after controlling for differences in the patient populations, researchers found that the 2008 cohort had significantly lower prevalence of dementia. So while numbers of people living with dementia (PLWD) are rising as the older population increases, the proportion of older people living with the disease is falling. This they attribute to public health campaigning and the mediating effects of cardiovascular disease, provoked by smoking, poor diet and low exercise.

Very few of the narratives that have been covered so far talk to dementia and vulnerability. Overall (2003) has been careful to say that prolongivism 'works' as a concept, so long as people continue the capacity for emotion, perception, thought and action. Narratives of active and productive ageing tend to shunt vulnerability into the twilight of the fourth age. This fourth age, following a third age of active engagement, can, in the words of Gilleard and Higgs (2013) 'better be understood as representative of 'an ascribed community of otherness, set apart from the everyday experiences and practices of later life' (2013: 370). Dementia, in particular, is seen as something threatening that disqualifies people from social engagement and makes them unable to compete in the market (Ritchie et al., 2015). Spirituality values the vulnerability of old age and of the small proportion of older adults who experience dementia, as a common element of humanity. However, apart from a few exceptions (MacKinlay, 2001; Swinton & Pattison, 2010; Mowat & O'Neill, 2013), this relationship is underexplored.

While it leaves the purpose of a long life open, anti-ageing medicine intends to avoid ageing by extending and enhancing the adult lifecourse. It taps into narratives that focus on the maintenance of hope and personal continuity. Dementia, however, teaches us to manage decline in the absence of a clear cure. It connects us to negative discontinuity. In the absence of that hope, so important to medical optimism, people with dementia are often perceived as a reminder of hopelessness, evoking various distancing strategies, such as simply managing an unresponsive body or more benignly as a puzzle to be understood (Carr & Biggs, 2017). The person living with dementia (PLWD) is othered, leaving the possibilities for empathy and engagement increasingly remote.

If dementia is not seen as a disease, but as a normal part of ageing, it sets up a significant tension based on early understandings of senility and senescence as an inevitable process, affecting wider public perceptions of later life. Seeing it as a disease, as an intrusion into, but external to, self-identity sets up a parallel set of tensions. An approach based on person-centred care includes a moral obligation to search for the other's identity and interdependence in a growing absence of reciprocity. Do we, then, intergenerationally speaking, concentrate on the otherness of the other and try to understand it or attempt to recognise the similarities between people with and without dementia or some place in between? The perception of

PLWD as vulnerable and inarticulate victims of a disease has led to policy focusing on the protective regulation of care environments, while the growing voice of activists with dementia themselves to the development of dementia-friendly public environments. If, as medical science continues to promise, greater understanding of disease processes will provide a cure, then this debate will become an 'as-if' thought experiment. How would we relate to the other in a relationship that is increasingly non-reciprocal? What are the limits and the prerequisites of personhood? How should society respond to vulnerability in old age? Until then, the presence of dementia in the public mind requires critical analysis.

Dementia in the public domain

In public perception, Dementia acts as an extreme case of the fear of ageing as well as existing as a phenomenon in its own right. Ballenger (2006), for example, claims that 'senile dementia seems to taint the entire experience of ageing. In its relentless inevitability, deeply associated with ageing and the mere passage of time, it makes a mockery of the achievement of longevity' (2006: 107).

According to Scodellaro and Pin's (2013) review of studies in English and in French, dementia and ageing have become blurred and their relationship ambiguous. Dementia appears as something that has become a leading narrative for ageing more generally, disqualifying personal, social and economic investment in the old. Leon et al. (2015) have found, during a period of extensive campaigning, between 2008 and 2013, there were only minor changes in this association and attitudes to dementia among the general public. Respondents were more likely to put it in the three most serious diseases facing society (the others being AIDS and cancer) with close family carers having a keener sense of seriousness. In a systematic review of the literature on public knowledge of dementia (Cahill et al., 2015), the majority of studies consistently found only fair to moderate understanding by the general public, with the most common misconception that dementia was a normal part of ageing. Knowledge of dementia was reported to be less among racial and ethnic minority groups than in majority populations.

Social images associated with dementia range from the relatively benign attempts to portray waves eroding messages on a beach, trees with falling leaves and erasers at work on personal portraits to floods, wars and evocations of the living dead. Popular newspapers may focus on the extraordinary and calamitous destruction of former celebrities' selves and their embattled carers. Even high-end journals, such as the *Financial Review* (Jay, 2015: June), are not immune to signs of moral panic, reporting 'feral' elders, whose aggressive behaviours constituted a threat to care staff and indicate institutional failure.

The contingency of public perception and its social construction is perhaps most clearly indicated by historical study. Mediaeval understandings of memory and memory loss foregrounded a timeless soul as a background to self. Here, memory was secondary and identity dependent on the possibilities for future salvation. Katz (2013) argues that such comparative approaches question the importance of remembering as an anchor for identity and what its function might be. However, with the development of industrial society, persons such as Beard (1874) began to use senility in a struggle for generational ascendency. In his book *Legal Responsibility in Old Age*, Beard states that 'men die as trees die . . . slowly and frequently from the top first'. Senility is portrayed as a social ill requiring the transfer of assets and power from the old (or what we might now consider later middle age) to the young. Zelig (2014) has associated a modern history of dementia with an increasing frequency of metaphors of such as tsunamis, as an unstoppable destructive force. George and Whitehouse (2014) have connected the parallel development of a war on terror, a war on Alzheimer's, and associations of homeland threat. Both show the ability of metaphor to mutate depending on the perceived threat of the day. It is as if, once labelled, living with dementia becomes opened to surveillance and its assumed blankness becomes a screen on which social anxieties can be projected.

Perhaps most potent and enduring is an association between the supposed behaviour of zombies and the social space created for dementia (Behuniak, 2013). In emotional-psychological terms, both are connected with horror: disgust at decay and a fear of being devoured. In behavioural terms, associations draw on shuffling, incoherent groaning, while in social terms, both are portrayed as a threat that is relentless and ultimately overwhelming, a seeming loss of self and the ability to recognise others other than to consume them. She calls this a 'dehumanisation based on disgust and terror' leading to 'a politics of revulsion and fear' (Behuniak, 2013: 70). Zelig (2014) takes this further, connecting anxiety about old age and mental illness with the politics of individualism and social disintegration created by voracious capitalism, which we simultaneously have to live with and distance ourselves from. These processes are not so much seen as a metaphor, explaining dementia to the uninitiated; rather, they create a narrative space in which the two images – zombies and people living with dementia – become merged, until they are almost indistinguishable in their psychological and social meaning. It generates a process of delegitimisation by inclusion, into an extreme constellation of negative categories that feed from each other – relentless, consuming, stripped of personality, and dangerous, something that was us and whose stigma can contaminate by close association.

Perhaps unsurprisingly, Behuniak's 'Zombie' paper has collected a significant amount of Internet hits. The association lends a sort of freakish fascination from popular culture that makes dementia almost glamourous, were it not for its dehumanising properties and its amplification of otherness. The association reinforces the importance of the public sphere for ethical implications of perception and portrayal (Gerritsen, Oyebode & Gove, 2016) and the possibilities for intergenerational empathy in public debate (Haapala & Biggs, 2017).

Dementia as disease

So how have groups with an interest in dementia managed its relationship with social narratives, professional behaviour and personal identity?

The association between dementia and disease is powerful at a number of levels and arose from an alliance of health professionals, carers and concerned organisations in the United States during the 1970s. Fox (1989) has charted the rise of the Alzheimer's disease (AD) movement in the United States, pointing out that the development of a disease entity was not a natural or inevitable association, but the product of sustained political lobbying. AD, as 'a unifying construct provided a focus for political action', which led to the formation of the National Institute on Ageing and the release of resources for clinical research. A focus on the disease element of dementia served to separate it from specific age criteria, and Alzheimer's disease, in particular, came to symbolise a separation between normal and abnormal ageing. In an ironic twist of fate, Alzheimer's original and at the time largely overlooked work, which was not on senile (old age) but 'pre-senile' dementia, had led to a renewed and progressive distinction between disease and 'normal' ageing. By 1992, the WHO had adopted the following definition, emphasising cognitive degeneration caused by illness and having secondary effects:

> Dementia is a syndrome due to disease of the brain, usually of a chronic or progressive nature, in which there is disturbance of multiple higher cortical functions, including memory, thinking, orientation, comprehension, calculation, learning capacity, language, and judgement. Consciousness is not clouded. Impairments of cognitive function are commonly accompanied, and occasionally preceded, by deterioration in emotional control, social behaviour, or motivation.
>
> (World Health Organization, 1992)

By 2016, the WHO stated:

> dementia is a syndrome in which there is deterioration in memory, thinking, behaviour and the ability to perform everyday activities. Although dementia mainly affects older people, it is not a normal part of ageing. Dementia is one of the major causes of disability and dependency among older people worldwide. Dementia has physical, psychological, social and economical impact on caregivers, families and society'
>
> (World Health Organization, 2016)

Seeing dementia as principally a disease has not only rekindled hope of a cure; it has sparked initiatives internationally, such as the G8 initiative signed by G8 health and science ministers on 11 December 2013 (G8, 2013). This initiative set an ambition to identify a cure or a disease-modifying therapy for dementia by 2025. International momentum also resulted in a WHO Global Dementia Observatory in 2016.

The disease understanding of dementia means that it's not normal and PLWD not culpable. It's a containable threat. It's something we can be viewed to be doing something about. And under the guidance of the WHO, it has come to be seen not only as a neurodegenerative illness, provoked initially by the influence of US insurance eligibility criteria, but as a disability, opening the door to a wider discussion on rights and social attitudes.

Narratives arising from disease

While the promotion of dementia as a disease has had significant research, clinical and policy effects, Herskovits (1995) has argued that there is also a 'the loss of self' narrative linked to a medicalised and technical focus on brain dysfunction. Connecting a disease narrative to funding and legitimacy promises the possibility of creating order out of chaos, legitimising certain sites for intervention. The Alzheimer's disease movement, according to this view, has, like anti-ageing medicine, become part of Estes' (1979) 'aging enterprise' – a close connection between the interests health and other professionals and the development of new markets for research and products. A disease narrative also contains considerable ambivalence in so far as the PLWD can no longer be held responsible for their conduct. Hope of a cure, however, is maintained, lending new strength to medical practice.

Loss of agency has become a key issue in a struggle over definitions of disease and perceived threats to selfhood. Davis (2004) criticised the first WHO definition that identifies dementia as a cognitive process at the expense of understanding its social and emotional consequences. A medicalised narrative, he argues, presents ageing generally as a deviation from natural processes, which counters the advantages of seeing dementia exclusively as a disease. A link to memory loss also challenges the boundary between normality and pathology. Ballenger (2006), for example, argues that stigma associated with memory loss signifies a 'performance failure' for older adults in general. She claims that stigma associated with Alzheimer's disease throws the pathology solution for identity into disarray, defining stigma as 'the amount of anxiety surrounding the boundary between the normal and the pathological' (2006: 114). Beard and Neary (2013) refer here to a 'making sense of nonsense' in which people with mild cognitive impairment are 'often deemed incapable (and perhaps unworthy) of contributing to the social discourse surrounding their illness experience' (2013: 130). This predicament is made more complex by uncertainty over definitions of memory loss, the boundary between normal and abnormal forgetting plus ambiguity over the efficacy of treatment regimes. For example, the Lancet Neurology Commission (Winblad et al., 2016) indicated that 20% of diagnoses were in the absence of neuropathology at autopsy, while 33% exhibit high levels of neuropathology without any symptoms. Further, 50% of cases in a US study of 90 plus patients at autopsy found that people with dementia had not sufficient neuropathology to merit diagnosis on biomedical grounds (Corrada, Berlau & Kawas, 2012). In other words, one can have the neuropathology and not suffer from dementia and also not have the pathology and still get the symptoms.

PLWD's reactions to neuropathology itself can also create stigma that influences identity, which Scholl and Sabat (2008) attribute to reactions to the effects of neuropathology, interactions with the environment in which one lives, and how one is treated by others including service gatekeepers. More widely, older people may become sensitised to 'stereotype threat', an awareness of the stereotyping potential that ageing holds in the minds of others, which itself negatively affects the older person's performance (Scholl & Sabat, 2008). However, Beard and Fox

(2008) report that their respondents 'did not routinely perceive their experiences as pathological but rather were socialised into viewing age related forgetfulness as symbolic of disease' (2008: 1509). And while diagnosis can lead to social disenfranchisement and the label meant that one not only had to manage the manifestations of disease but also personal identity and social interactions with others, it nevertheless opened new possibilities for personal agency and impression management. Respondents actively used the label 'as a resource and as a phenomenon that needs to be incorporated into their self identity' (2008: 1509). It excused certain behaviours, occasioned humour (as the cartoon says, 'You accuse me of dementia? I'll forget that you said that' (Bartlett, 2013) and foregrounded other areas of competence. As such, dementia as a disease holds meaning that is both comforting and unnerving (Davis, 2004). Psychosocial tension surrounding stigma does not work well, for example, alongside medical advances that require increasingly early diagnosis. Early intervention can be experienced as the 'creep' of a disease narrative into normal everyday behaviour, which in this case increases the likelihood of identity threat.

Ambiguity is piled on ambiguity here as a disease narrative appears to simultaneously reinforce the boundary separating the senile from the rest of us, frees sufferers for responsibility for certain forms of conduct, opens private lives to surveillance and stigmatisation and yet offers new forms of agency and identity maintenance. But what also comes through is a certain confusion of voice. Who, in other words, is speaking, and what messages are being conveyed? The medical voice claims objectivity, hope and reconnection to the social order but is at root a third party, an observing position, located outside the personal experience of disease. It is speaking from the outside, whether as a professional helper, or as persons with dementia who can distance themselves from the disease itself.

Enter person-centred care

A disease narrative, while holding many advantages, also contains a tendency to ignore interpersonal relations and wider social inequalities as factors contributing to dementia. In this section, the first of these issues will be considered. A subsequent section will examine social inequality.

In order to understand both the dehumanising processes associated with traditional dementia care and provide an alternative, Kitwood (1997: 8) proposed 'a definition of personhood . . . It is a standing or status that is bestowed upon one human being, by others, in the context of relationship and social being. It implies recognition, respect and trust' (1997: 8).

His formulation, which proved crucial to the development of person-centred care, places special emphasis on relationships: 'To form and hold relationships, essential here is the ability to understand and identify with the interests, desires and needs of others' (1997: 9). Occasioning a shift from a third to a second person stance towards the person with dementia, Kitwood identifies two key elements in the power of meaningful interaction between paid carers and PLWD and the capacity of the former to empathise with the latter. In a sort of reverse question to Turing's 'is an unseen computer intelligent' test, he asks, however eroded the signals, can we still see the person? Kitwood's answer is to search harder and the person behind the dementia can still be reached. There is an element of ambiguity in Kitwood's formulation, however, in so far as his argument drifts between 'the moral agent and the subject of moral concern' (9), which he refers to as stronger and weaker forms of the same dilemma. So is he talking about a carer's capacities, the cared for's, or a combination of both? Also, if personhood is contingent upon relationship, then what happens if the capacity for relationship as reciprocity is severely eroded?

Kitwood presents two answers to this criticism: first, he maintains that contemporary relationships have been reduced to 'autonomy and rationality' by a form of 'extreme individualism in western societies', which then allows the dismissal of personhood in dementia. He argues that we should rather rely 'more strongly on feeling, emotion and the ability to live in relationships' (1997: 10) and on 'moral solidarity' and the essential unity of all human beings. Second, both Kitwood and Sabat and Harre (1992) argue that people with dementia are capable of meaning-making despite attacks on the components of memory and language. They maintain both a sense of selfhood and a desire to form relationships however much depleted. Indeed evidence from intergenerational dementia programmes indicates that type of programme is less important than meaningful and shared opportunities for relationship building (Galbraith et al., 2015). The problem is that systems of care fall subject to 'malignant social psychology' (Kitwood, 1990) or 'malignant positioning' (Sabat, 2003) whereby the PLWD is placed negatively by others and his or her humanity dismissed. The capacity of the person without dementia to empathise with the person living with it and resist the enveloping context of social ageism in general and fears of dementia in particular results, it is argued, in a de-othering of the other, who nevertheless becomes more difficult a focus of relationship and exchange. Kitwood placed dementia within a psychopolitical context, which is often overlooked. His approach has been interpreted as 'looking for the person' with a radical impact on practice, which has become mainstream in finding practical ways of improving services (Brooker, 2007).

Relationship as emotional labour

Davis (2004) has critiqued Kitwood's person-centred approach because it tasks formal carers, friends and family with a search for the remains of an eroded personal identity. He claims that whilst well-meaning, the approach is overly romantic in its expectations, setting carers up increasingly to fail as the disease progresses. This process of identity erosion has been identified as a transfer of self onto others (Herskovits, 1995) as relationships become increasingly less reciprocal. Here, Buse and Twigg (2016) refer to others as the 'holder' or 'curator' of identity, such that the carer is tasked with somehow keeping lost memories alive.

The second person position of caring generates ambivalent emotions. Kessler (2007, in Behuniak, 2013) sums up these feelings as 'when you spend your days around people with the disease, despite the amazing moments and the times you feel like Mother Theresa on meth, the mantra that runs through your head is: not me, not me, not me, please not me' (2013: 144).

Earlier literature is much more explicit, with Fontana and Smith (1989) remarking on the fear that dementia evokes of becoming oneself a victim, terrifying precisely because one can identify with the PLWD's situation. The impact of a dwindling reciprocity on sustaining shared meaning interlinks with a fear for one's own aged future. To work, the rewards here may be for a more abstract dimension than the rewards of the task itself; it is that of being saint-like, of being seen by others but principally oneself as being worthy (Ames, 2016). The erosion of reciprocal meaning-making throws one back on alternative sources of perseverance in the face of expectations that don't really work anymore.

Hochschild (1983) developed the concept of emotional labour to examine forms of work that rely principally on interpersonal relationships. She claims that such work generates 'feeling rules' that set up a tension between genuine emotional responses and expectations of caring behaviour tacitly scripted by the demands of the tasks at hand. Her original work concerned the behaviour of flight attendants and was extended to include working mothers and nurses (Smith, 1999). Emotional labour can require surface and deep acting including outward appearance or feeling work, which like method acting inhabits the beliefs and identity of the workers involved. The labour exists in bringing genuine feelings into line with occupational or commercial demands (Loewenthal, 2002), which Hochschild refers to as 'regulating emotional displays according to a set of occupational prescriptions' (1983: 33).

Emotional labour, it is argued, requires acts of self-enforced transformation that move beyond task performance to emotional performance. It becomes a form of soft regulation in which emotional responsibility for the other is amplified by demands that one feels as well as behaves in conformity with the caring task, whether this is intuitively felt or not. It is closely related to Menzies' (1959) work on defences against anxiety. Here, routinisation of care work, forced actions that are in spite of or occlude nurses' immediate caring reaction, creating a sort of reverse emotional labour. Intuitive caring behaviours need to be suppressed in the service of task performance, which, when added to the social construction of dementia as a personal and societal threat, acts as a permissor for instrumental behaviour. Care work may therefore require emotional identification with others or an escape into rigid regulation. A number of writers have evidenced such a tension in dementia care work (Lopez, 2007; Kontos, Miller & Mitchell, 2009; Bailey et al., 2015; Hunter, Hadjistavropoulos & Kaasalainen, 2016), where rule following and time constraints curtail and eventually institutionalise routinised behaviour.

Bailey et al.'s (2015) study of NHS 'unqualified' care assistants followed a government report on hospital services that were 'failing to respond to the needs of older people with care and compassion' Abraham (2011). The researchers found that caring roles constituted an 'attempt to provide personalised care for people whose cognitive degeneration renders conventional relationship building very difficult' (2015: 246). Best practice was found to blend professional distance and 'a situated form of empathy' in which care was 'not so much a matter of being closer to the individual who is ill but rather one of being close to the truth of that individual's current dilemma' which 'requires a balancing of emotional engagement and detachment'. They argue that in dementia work, commonly accepted assumptions of social interaction do not apply, emphasising the productive role of detachment in competent caring. Overidentification can create 'a dynamic of self-delusion arising from unreciprocated exchange which can be taken home into (carer's) own families and personal lives' (263).

Similarly, Carr and Biggs (2017) found two strategies in Australian not-for-profit care homes. One relied on routinised 'misrecognition' of the caring task, where reporting and monitoring became attempts to avoid interaction with residents. A second, more adaptive strategy found workers seeing residents with advanced dementia as 'a puzzle'. Workers balanced the often erratic and unpredictable behaviour of residents with continued relationships by seeing interactions as puzzles to be solved. This formed a means of mediating the relationship, seeing changes and behaviour in a positive light and offering an imaginative space that can incorporate uncertainty and a degree of understanding. The authors suggest that the puzzle approach combines empathy, professional distance and a form of problem-solving creativity.

These naturally occurring strategies parallel Beard and Fox's (2008) attempts to re-name PLWD as 'forgetful people'. Using forgetfulness or absent-mindedness has also been prominent in Japanese campaigning, where 'chi-ho' has been replaced by 'ninchisho', from associations with shameful foolishness to absent-mindedness (Miyamoto, George & Whitehouse, 2011). The Finnish organisation Muistiliitto (2017) also refers to memory loss rather than disease, with a play on words *Välitä Muista*, meaning both remembering and care for others.

What emerges from these studies is a reminder that emotional labour and person-centred care are not necessarily incompatible if a balance can be struck between professional distance and interpersonal empathy, albeit under difficult relational conditions.

One is reminded there that health and caring establishments are workplaces as well as places where people are trying to live their daily, homelike lives. Problems arise when working conditions have themselves been eroded to a point where empathic engagement is almost impossible. A series of contradictory positions then intersect in the performance of care roles. Johnson's (2015) case study of nursing care indicates, for example, that

> carers, encouraged by the company, naturalised their emotional labour, and that this had contradictory consequences. On the one hand it justified the economic devaluation of the carer's work and left her vulnerable to emotional over-involvement and client aggression. On the other, it allowed the worker to defend the moral interests of those within her care and see when those interests were in in conflict with the economic motivations of her employer.
> (2015: 112)

Hunter et al. (2016) note the tensions created by combining relationship and an intrinsic motivation to care with cultures that emphasise short-term time economic efficiencies rather than long-term solutions to difficult problems. They argue that a tension exists between 'efficiency' and personal care, resulting in a stripping back of non-tending elements (such as building relationships) of paid care in the interests of economy and a daily balancing act between transparency and deception. Lopez's (2007) ethnographic study connects depersonalised care with wider funding and regulatory regimes. He observed contradictions between the regulatory requirements of the job, time allowed for task performance and poor staff ratios, a combination that made rule breaking a necessary part of care work. He points out that in the United States, 'no levels of staffing supported by the current federal reimbursement system would allow nurse aides to actually live up to official care standards' (2007: 241). Canadian researchers, Banerjee et al. (2012) report high levels of resident on carer abuse in such settings, which bear a close resemblance to forms of institutionalised 'social abuse' as discussed by Mysyuk et al. (2015). Banerjee et al. (2015) note the absence of the voice of care workers, which is hidden by routinised, task-based, 'assembly-line' activities, 'accountability, enacted as counting and documenting' (2015: 28), that took time away from the performance of care. Lopez (2007) points to collusive systems where managers tacitly acknowledge the problem but feeling powerless themselves, offer training responses, which give the impression of compliance, for example, lifting and getting up in the morning, but fail to address underlying structural failures. Under such conditions, institutionalised rule breaking creates a strategy to individualise care, where full compliance would constrain an ability to adopt principles of person-directed care (Kontos et al., 2009). Flexibility when rules don't work, however, is accompanied by anxiety and emotional labour when workers need to cover up. Such 'overlooking', if rules are worked round, attempts a rebalancing, but also avoids effective change.

These reports identify contradictions between contemporary economics of care, emotional labour and the principles of person-centred care. They also identify the mirroring of relational dynamics throughout organisational systems (Miller & Gwynne, 1972). In this case, emotional tensions, if unchecked by psychosocial understanding and supervision, can reflect themselves up and down a system of dementia care. Thus, the dehumanising tendencies of public attitudes interconnect with the experience of people with dementia, the conduct and treatment of care staff and the prioritising of instrumental rather than relational regimes. The needs of people with dementia, their carers and services become 'forgotten' in a system that emerges as routinised and time-poor. The erosion of the possibilities for reciprocity is mirrored in a denying and unresponsive system, which Davenhill (1998) argues is connected to deep-seated unconscious processes affecting public debate.

Eroded services that mirror public attitudes to dementia also intersect with multiple forms of jeopardy associated with social inequality. This may be particularly salient for those in a relationship of informal care.

Structural factors, risk and social inequality

Much has been made of the structural costs of dementia and of population ageing (OECD, 2015). National fiscal policies have largely responded by attempting to transfer risk from the public purse to private responsibility, even though this is already heavily weighted towards family and informal care rather than national economies. As much as 80% of the economic cost of dementia comes from indirect costs, consisting of about 40% each from social and informal care and only roughly 20% from direct medical costs (Prince et al., 2015). Indirect costs are carried by by unpaid, informal care provided by family members and friends, most often by spouses, daughters and daughters-in-law. The cost of caring is especially felt among low-income groups and in disadvantaged areas (Xiao et al., 2014; Ervin et al., 2015; Winblad et al., 2016). Time away from work leads to lost income, and caring work leads to increased levels of stress-related disorders and depression among the informal caregivers (van den Lee et al., 2017). Nair, Mansfield and Waller (2016) add that 'carers experience high rates of anxiety and depression, poorer physical health, financial pressures, and changes in employment'. With younger onset dementia, carers may be adolescents caring for a parent (Hutchinson et al., 2016). Data from low- and middle-income countries show that 94% of the care of people living with dementia is of the informal type, i.e., it is provided at home by the next of kin, while in high-income countries, this constitutes 66% (Wimo & Prince, 2010). Within countries, the risk of dementia is higher in low-income groups and population sub-groups living in disadvantaged areas, due to a higher prevalence of cardiovascular risk factors in dietary intake, obesity, depression, lack of physical activity, smoking, lack of social participation and low educational level and reduced access to care (Ervin et al., 2015; Wright et al., 2016; Winblad et al., 2016). Risk factors are also higher in rural than in urban areas (AIWH, 2010; Renehan et al., 2012). Living close to major roads can also increase risk (Chen et al., 2017).

Following a European Parliament (2013) report on people with dementia in the workplace, Ritchie et al. (2015) point out that changes to pension age eligibility plus earlier diagnosis will combine to identify more people with dementia in employment for whom supports would be needed. Bentham and La Fontaine (2007) point out that early symptoms are most likely to be noticed first in workplaces and have resulted in redundancy or dismissal for incompetence. Reasons, according to an Alzheimer's Australia report (2007), include problems with memory, word finding, learning new material, visual spatial tasks and concentration, plus reduced motivation. Despite campaigns, for example, in Finland (Alzheimer Europe, 2016) and the United Kingdom (ACAS, 2016), recognition and support for dementia in the workplace has, at the time of writing, been minimal.

So, socioeconomically disadvantaged groups within high- and lower-income countries are at higher risk of Alzheimer's disease. Caregivers in these families will be multiply-jeopardised, because most often, they are women, older adults, suffering from a chronic condition, and with a lower level of education and employment. If PLWD wish to stay at work, they face prejudice and disadvantage. When taken together, structural inequalities reflect back on the life quality of care workers, informal carers and those living with dementia themselves. It would appear that a public othering of PLWD ricochets within societies, interconnecting third- and second-person positioning. A final section examines the growing role of first-person voices and the experience of dementia itself.

First-person experiences of dementia

One of the continuing issues with forms of second-person relations, relating to dementia as a non-dementing person, is that it becomes difficult to identify the authentic voice of PLWD. Proxy voices stream into the vacuum, be that through state-based regulation, professional discourse or care provider activity, each of which may claim privileged knowledge to speak for vulnerable others (Carr & Biggs, 2017).

Bender and Cheston's (1997) work is perhaps exceptional in its early attempt to access 'the internal world of the dementia sufferer' (1997: 513). They report feelings engendered by the process of dementia in people 'anxious to what is happening and what will happen', including 'anxiety, depression, grief, despair, terror' (515). They suggest a shift in therapeutic understanding away from cognition and remembering to immediacy and emotion, also reflected in Herskovits' (1995) more positive evocation, that 'I can remember you with my heart'. Beard and Fox (2008) report that 'diagnosed individuals consciously navigated between the everyday experiences requiring innovative and fleeting management techniques and the stationary, technical jargon and explanatory frameworks of bio-medicine' (2008: 1518). Diagnosis can, they claim, 'simultaneously rob individuals of their unique attributes and serve to solidify group identity among those sharing common circumstances' (1518).

Many of the studies attempting to access experience have been qualitative, with small numbers of respondents. MacRae (2010) reports that PLWD resisted negative stereotyping with a determination to 'make the best of it'. Strategies such as humour, normalisation, present-time orientation and life review were used to create a meaningful life experience. The ability to live positively in the face of negative stereotyping has been a common strategy reported by PLWD and their carers (van Gennip et al., 2014). Weaks, Wilkinson and McLeod (2015) found particular challenges for PLWD and their families in telling others. Findings suggested that participants recognised the need to tell others about their diagnosis, but these conversations were difficult to initiate and manage and hindered the processing of emotions. Steeman et al. (2013), using depth interviewing, found that people with dementia experienced a tension between self-protecting and self-adjusting strategies. Dementia was seen as a threat to security and autonomy and an ability to retain meaningful membership of society. In more advanced stages, PLWDs' experiences may be positive due to decreased awareness hindering an acknowledgement of the negative, but the positivity can also serve as a façade to mask an inability or unwillingness to discuss fears concerning becoming a burden on others, being put into care and of losing one's mind. Following a review of social and cultural responses to living with dementia, Hulko (2009: 138) concludes that

> we cannot say there is one experience; rather there are a multitude of experiences that reflect the degree of privilege and oppression to which people with dementia are subject, based on their gender, 'racial', ethnic, and class backgrounds – that is, irrespective of their shared status as persons living with dementia.

For lower socioeconomic groups, things that they tended to forget 'really were not that important'; rather, emphasis was placed on the loss of practical day-to-day living skills, such as shopping, cooking and paying bills. For higher groups, loss of status and threats to autonomy and of marginalisation predominated. For lower groups, dementia became 'one more hurdle to overcome', whereas for higher-status groups, it became a significant threat to identity. De Boer et al. (2012) found that people in the early stages of dementia were very capable of sharing their experiences, often becoming more open and talkative in the course of an interview. For participants, thinking about the future involved an ongoing process of balancing feelings of fear and hope, but the overall tendency among this group was to try to live one day at a time and avoid worrying about the future.

Together, these studies indicate that people with dementia are active agents, who do not passively suffer the consequences of having dementia: they interact with their illness, their families and their carers.

Rights-based approaches

It is perhaps unsurprising, given experiential evidence of continued agency and psychosocial engagement, that increasing numbers of PLWD have adopted a rights-based approach. Bartlett (2014) reports on how activism and campaigning can relocate individuals' identities within the realm of work, through public speaking and other forms of participation. This adds to an identity of active citizenship but can come at a cost. 'Individuals may experience fatigue due to the dementia, and oppression linked to normative expectations about what someone with dementia "should" be like' (2014: 1299). Living positively, she says, is challenged by negative attitudes and accusations of being a fraud if the stereotype is not confirmed. Swaffer (2015), a dementia activist, has railed against the 'prescribed disengagement' that her physician recommended. Instead of preparing for a withdrawal from society, Swaffer encourages PLWD to see it as a disability and ask for support at work and at home and to define themselves by identities and skills other than dementia. Swaffer has been active in expanding the US-based Dementia Alliance International (DAI), which offers exclusive membership to people with dementia, and the European Working Group of People with Dementia (EWGPD). Both of these organisations promote a 'nothing about us, without us' approach to policy and practice and draw on the experience of the wider disability movement for inspiration. The Australian DAI, for example, provides weekly online support groups for people with dementia; 24-hour/day online zoom chat rooms are also available for a number of different groups, including an exclusive zoom room for people with dementia and one for family and care partners, plus members of the LGBTI community. This arrangement obviates a sensitivity to different perspectives based on relationship and identity. Both DAI and EWDPD make regular submissions to government. They represent a significant shift in strategic thinking around the rights of older adults that has been reflected in the United Nations Working Group on Older People's call for dementia to be seen principally as a disability, rather than a disease. While debate on the competing voices of patients, carers and workers are common in other discourses on disability (Beresford, 2013; Wiersma et al., 2016), in dementia, it has been less quick to develop. It is sometimes, as Beresford warns, difficult to discern which constituency is being heard and who is speaking for whom. This is further complicated because people can live with dementia in different forms and stages. It may also reflect a tendency for caring organisations and government agencies to take a protective role towards people with dementia, plus stigmatising assumptions that dementia is an all-or-nothing experience rather than a continuum.

Concluding comments

Dementia, then, is presented as threatening the promise of a long life and as the great fear lurking within it. However, as the numbers of older adults grow and even though the likelihood of having dementia is declining, more people with the condition will need to be included into society. Popular culture and by degrees medical practice, as third-person discourses, have placed people with dementia in the position of the 'age-other' and dementia as the discontinuity that none wish to experience. Dementia exemplifies within-age thinking, in so far as attempts are made to split the experience away from other age groups, or parts of the ageing self that are considered diseased. There has been little between-age thinking as the experience has become estranged from other elements of identity. Indeed, dementia presents a kaleidoscope of increasing present-centredness, as reflected in the experience itself, and lifetime-centredness as it becomes associated more generally with adult ageing, especially in others. This 'not me' narrative has, historically speaking, had the unfortunate effect of eclipsing the first-person voice and associated rights-based approaches that had become characteristic of disability and mental health survivor movements. Intergenerationally, overcoming fear plus normalising interpersonal relations appear twin priorities. Relations between self and other and the possibilities for empathy, while challenging, are evidenced by emerging strategies for person-centredness, negotiated emotional reciprocity, rights-based approaches and workplace-based sites of engagement. Future development may require a closer attention to the intergenerational because dementia is an age-inflected association and because care often takes place between persons of different age groups and is therefore stratified by age. Dementia care, whether in community, residential or hospital settings, involves the resolution of contradictions between the workplace and lived-in private spaces and the development of dementia-friendly environments. A cultural shift is suggested, then, from the fascinated or sensationalising observer to the challenges of connection and reciprocity. In a best-case scenario, dementia becomes a puzzle leading to co-creation and shared problem solving. In a worst-case scenario, it becomes an extreme case of the commodification of emotional labour and a specific instance of attempts to estrange us from the promise of a long life.

References

Abraham, A. (2011). Care and compassion? Report of the health service ombudsman on ten investigations into NHS care of older people. Parliamentary and Health Service Ombudsman, London, United Kingdom. Retrieved from www.ombudsman.org.uk/__data/assets/pdf_

ACAS. (2016). Dealing with dementia in the workplace. Advisory, Conciliation and Arbitration Service, Worksite Snippets 2015. Retrieved April 17, 2016, from www.acas.org.uk/index.aspx?articleid=5429

AIWH. (2010). Australian institute of health and welfare, Australia's health 2010. Australia's health series no. 12. Canberra, ACT: Author.

Alzheimer Europe. (2016). National dementia strategies: Finland. Retrieved July 29, 2016, from www.alzheimer-europe.org/Policy-in-Practice2/National-Dementia-Strategies/Finland#fragment1

Alzheimer's Australia. (2007). Exploring the needs of younger people with dementia in Australia. Retrieved July 29, 2016, from www.fightdementia.org.au/services/further-reading-and-resources.aspx

Ames, S. (2016). What happens to the person with dementia? *Journal of Religion, Spirituality & Aging, 28*(1–2), 118–135.

Bailey, S., Scales, K., Lloyd, J., Schneider, J., & Jones, R. (2015). The emotional labour of health-care assistants in inpatient dementia care. *Ageing and Society, 35*(2), 246–269.

Ballenger, J. F. (2006). The biomedical deconstruction of senility and the persistent stigmatization of old age in the United States. In A. Leibing & L. Cohen (Eds.), *Thinking about dementia: Culture, loss, and the anthropology of senility* (pp. 106–120). New Brunswick, NJ: Rutgers University Press.

Banerjee, A., Armstrong, P., Daly, T., Armstrong, H., & Braedley, S. (2015). "Careworkers don't have a voice": Epistemological violence in residential care for older people. *Journal of Aging Studies, 33*, 28–36.

Banerjee, A., Daly, T., Armstrong, P., Szebehely, M., Armstrong, H., & Lafrance, S. (2012). Structural violence in long-term, residential care for older people: Comparing Canada and Scandinavia. *Social Science & Medicine, 74*(3), 390–398.

Bartlett, R. (2013). Playing with meaning: Using cartoons to disseminate research findings. *Qualitative Research, 13*(2), 214–227.

Bartlett, R. (2014). Citizenship in action: The lived experiences of citizens with dementia who campaign for social change. *Disability & Society, 29*(8), 1291–1304.

Beard, G. M. (1874). *Legal responsibility in old age.* New York, NY: Russells.

Beard, R. L., & Fox, P. J. (2008). Resisting social disenfranchisement: Negotiating collective identities and everyday life with memory loss. *Social Science & Medicine, 66*(7), 1509–1520.

Beard, R. L., & Neary, T. M. (2013). Making sense of nonsense: Experiences of mild cognitive impairment. *Sociology of Health & Illness, 35*(1), 130–146.

Behuniak, S. (2013). The living dead? The construction of people with Alzheimer's disease as zombies. *Ageing and Society, 31*(1), 70–92.

Bender, M. P., & Cheston, R. (1997). Inhabitants of a lost kingdom: A model of the subjective experiences of dementia. *Ageing & Society, 17*(5), 513–532.

Bentham, P., & La Fontaine, J. (2007). Service development for younger people with dementia. *Psychiatry, 7*(2), 84–87.

Beresford, P. (2013). Developments in mental health policy and practice: Service user critiques. In J. Swain, S. French, C. Barnes & C. Thomas (Eds.), *Disabling barriers-enabling environments.* (pp. 262–269) London, UK: Sage.

Brooker, D. (2007). *Person centred dementia care*. Bradford: University of Bradford Press.

Buse, C., & Twigg, J. (2016). Materialising memories: Exploring the stories of people with dementia through dress. *Ageing and Society, 36*(6), 1115–1135.

Cahill, S., Pierce, M., Werner, P., Darley, A., & Bobersky, A. (2015). A systematic review of the public's knowledge and understanding of Alzheimer's disease and dementia. *Alzheimer Disease & Associated Disorders, 29*(3), 255–275.

Carr, A., & Biggs, S. (2017). Exploring regulatory clusters in dementia care. Research Insight 3. Melbourne, Australia: Brotherhood of St Laurence. Retrieved from www.bsl. org.au/knowledge/browse-publications/exploring-regulatory-clusters-in-dementia-care/

Chen, H., Kwong, J. C., Copes, R., Tu, K., Villeneuve, P. J., van Donkelaar, A., . . . Wilton, A. S. (2017). Living near major roads and the incidence of dementia, Parkinson's disease, and multiple sclerosis: A population-based cohort study. *The Lancet, 389*(10070), 718–726.

Corrada, M. M., Berlau, D. J., & Kawas, C. H. (2012). A population-based clinicopathological study in the oldest-old: The 90+ study. *Current Alzheimer Research, 9*, 709–717.

Davenhill, R. (1998). No truce with the furies. *Journal of Social Work Practice, 12*(2), 149–157.

Davis, D. H. (2004). Dementia: Sociological and philosophical constructions. *Social Science & Medicine, 58*(2), 369–378.

de Boer, M. E., Dröes, R. M., Jonker, C., Eefsting, J. A., & Hertogh, C. M. (2012). Thoughts on the future: The perspectives of elderly people with early-stage Alzheimer's disease and the implications for advance care planning. *AJOB Primary Research, 3*(1), 14–22.

Ervin, K., Pallant, J., Terry, D. F., Bourke, L., Pierce, D., & Glenister, K. (2015). A descriptive study of health, lifestyle and sociodemographic characteristics and their relationship to known dementia risk factors in rural Victorian communities. *AIMS Medical Science, 2*(3), 246–260. DOI:10.3934/medsci.2015.3.246

Estes, C. L. (1979). *The aging enterprise*. San Francisco, CA: Jossey-Bass.

European Parliament. (2013). Neurodegenerative diseases in the workplace. Retrieved from www.europarl.europa.eu/RegData/bibliotheque/briefing/2013/130580/ LDM_BRI(2013)130580_REV1_EN.pdf

Fontana, A., & Smith, R. W. (1989). Alzheimer's disease victims: The "unbecoming" of self and the normalization of competence. *Sociological Perspectives, 32*(1), 35–46.

Fox, P. (1989). From senility to Alzheimer's disease: The rise of the Alzheimer's disease movement. *The Milbank Quarterly, 67*(1), 58–102.

G8 Health and Science Ministers. (2013, December 11). G8 dementia summit declaration. Retrieved July 29, 2016, from www.gov.uk/government/publications/g8-dementia-summit-agreements/g8-dementia-summit-declaration

Galbraith, B., Larkin, H., Moorhouse, A., & Oomen, T. (2015). Intergenerational programs for persons with dementia: A scoping review. *Journal of Gerontological Social Work, 58*(4), 357–378.

George, D., & Whitehouse, P. (2014). The war (on terror) on Alzheimer's. *Dementia, 13*(1), 120–130.

Gerritsen, D. L., Oyebode, J., & Gove, D. (2016, June 10). Ethical implications of the perception and portrayal of dementia. *Dementia*, London. DOI:10.1177/1471301216654036

Gilleard, C., & Higgs, P. (2013). The fourth age and the concept of a "social imaginary": A theoretical excursus. *Journal of Aging Studies, 27*(4), 368–376.

Haapala, I. & Biggs, S. (2017). Generational intelligence and dementia in the public domain. In G. MacDonald (Ed.), *Reframing dementia as a social and cultural experience* (pp. 109–120). New York: Springer.

Hebert, L. E., Weuve, J., Scherr, P. A., & Evans, D. A. (2013). Alzheimer disease in the United States (2010–2050) estimated using the 2010 census. *Neurology, 80*(19), 1778–1783.

Herskovits, E. (1995). Struggling over subjectivity: Debates about the "self" and Alzheimer's disease. *Medical Anthropology Quarterly, 9*(2), 146–164.

Hochschild, A. (1983). *The managed heart: Commercialization of human feeling.* Berkeley, CA: University of California Press.

Hulko, W. (2009). From "not a big deal" to "hellish": Experiences of older people with dementia. *Journal of Aging Studies, 23*(3), 131–144.

Hunter, P. V., Hadjistavropoulos, T., & Kaasalainen, S. (2016). A qualitative study of nursing assistants' awareness of person-centred approaches to dementia care. *Ageing and Society, 36*(6), 1211–1237.

Hutchinson, K., Roberts, C., Daly, M., Bulsara, C., & Kurrle, S. (2016). Empowerment of young people who have a parent living with dementia: A social model perspective. *International Psychogeriatrics, 28*(4), 657–668. DOI:10.1017/S1041610215001714

Jay, C. (2015, June 10). Dementia troublemakers problem in retirement homes. *Financial Review*. Retrieved October 7, 2016, from www.afr.com/news/politics/national/dementia-troublemakers-problem-in-retirement-homes-20150610-ghknnu

Johnson, E. K. (2015). The business of care: The moral labour of care workers. *Sociology of Health & Illness, 37*(1), 112–126.

Katz, S. (2013). Dementia, personhood and embodiment: What can we learn from the medieval history of memory? *Dementia, 12*(3), 303–314.

Kessler, L. (2007). *Dancing with Rose: Finding life in the land of Alzheimer's.* New York, NY: Viking.

Kitwood, T. (1990). The dialectics of dementia: With particular reference to Alzheimer's disease. *Ageing and Society, 10*(2), 177–196.

Kitwood, T. (1997). *Dementia reconsidered: The person comes first.* Buckingham, England: Open University Press.

Kontos, P. C., Miller, K. L., & Mitchell, G. J. (2009). Neglecting the importance of the decision making and care regimes of personal support workers: A critique of standardization of care planning through the RAI/MDS. *The Gerontologist, 50*(3), 352–362.

Leon, C., Pin, S., Kreft-Jais, C., & Arwidson, P. (2015). Perceptions of Alzheimer's disease in the French population. *Journal of Alzheimer's Disease, 47*, 467–478.

Loewenthal, D. (2002). Involvement and emotional labour. *Soundings, 17*, 151–162.

Lopez, S. H. (2007). Efficiency and the fix revisited: Informal relations and mock routinization in a nonprofit nursing home. *Qualitative Sociology, 30*, 225–247.

MacKinlay, E. (2001). *The spiritual dimension of ageing.* London, England: Jessica Kingsley Publishers.

MacRae, H. (2010). Managing identity while living with Alzheimer's disease. *Qualitative Health Research, 20*(3), 293–305.

Matthews, F. E., Arthur, A., Barnes, L. E., Bond, J., Jagger, C., Robinson, L., & Medical Research Council Cognitive Function and Ageing Collaboration. (2013). A two-decade comparison of prevalence of dementia in individuals aged 65 years and older from three geographical areas of England: Results of the cognitive function and ageing study I and II. *The Lancet, 382*(9902), 1405–1412.

Menzies, I. (1959). *Social systems as a defence against anxiety.* London, England: Tavistock.

Miller, E. J., & Gwynne, G. V. (1972). *A life apart.* London, England: Tavistock.

Miyamoto, M., George, D. R., & Whitehouse, P. J. (2011). Government, professional and public efforts in Japan to change the designation of dementia (chihō). *Dementia, 10*(4), 475–486.

Mowat, H., & O'Neill, M. (2013, January 14). Spirituality and ageing: Implications for the care and support of older people. *IRISS Insights*, *19*. Retrieved July 30, 2016, from www.iriss.org.uk/resources/insights/spirituality-ageing-implications-care-support-older-people

Mysyuk, Y., Westendorp, R. G. J., Biggs, S., & Lindenberg, J. (2015). Listening to the voices of abused older people: Should we classify system abuse? *BMJ: British Medical Journal (Online)*, *350*, h2697.

Nair, B., Mansfield, E., & Waller, A. (2016). A race against time: The dementia epidemic. *Archives of Medicine and Health Sciences*, *4*(1), 127–134.

OECD. (2015, March 13). Addressing dementia. The OECD Response. OECD Health Policy Studies. Retrieved July 28, 2016, from www.oecd.org/health/addressing-dementia-9789264231726-en.htm

Overall, C. (2003). *Aging, death & human longevity*. Berkeley, LA: California University Press.

Prince, M., Knapp, M., Guerchet, M., McCrone, P., Prina, M., Comas-Herrera, A., . . . Salimkumar, D. (2014). *Dementia UK: Update* (2nd ed.). London, UK: Alzheimer's Society.

Prince, M., Wimo, A., Guerchet, M., Ali, G.-C., Wu, Y.-T., Prina, M., & Alzheimer's Disease International. (2015). *World Alzheimer report 2015: The global impact of dementia: An analysis of prevalence, incidence, cost and trends*. London, UK: Alzheimer's Disease International.

Renehan, E., Dow, B., Lin, X., Blackberry, I., Haapala, I., Gaffy, E., . . . Hendy, S. (2012, July). Healthy ageing literature review. Report for the Victorian Government, Department of Health, Wellbeing, Integrated Care and Ageing Division. Melbourne: Victorian Government.

Ritchie, L., Banks, P., Danson, M., Tolson, D., & Borrowman, F. (2015). Dementia in the workplace: A review. *Journal of Public Mental Health*, *14*(1), 24–34.

Sabat, S. R. (2003). Malignant positioning and the predicament of people with Alzheimer's disease. In R. Harré & F. M.Moghaddam (Eds.), *The self and others: Positioning individuals and groups in personal, political, and cultural contexts* (pp. 85–98). Westport, CT: Praeger.

Sabat, S. R., & Harre, R. (1992). The construction and deconstruction of self in Alzheimer's disease. *Ageing & Society*, *12*(4), 443–461.

Scholl, J. M., & Sabat, S. R. (2008). Stereotypes, stereotype threat and ageing: Implications for the understanding and treatment of people with Alzheimer's disease. *Ageing and Society*, *28*(1), 103–130.

Scodellaro, C., & Pin, S. (2013). The ambiguous relationships between ageing and Alzheimer's disease: A critical literature review. *Dementia*, *12*(1), 137–151.

Smith, P. (1999). Logging emotions. *Soundings*, *11*, 128–137.

Steeman, E. S., Tournoy, J., Grypdonck, M., Godderis, J., & Dierckx de Casterlé, B. (2013). Managing identity in early-stage dementia: Maintaining a sense of being valued. *Ageing and Society*, *33*, 216–242.

Swaffer, K. (2015). Dementia and prescribed disengagement™. *Dementia*, *14*(1), 3–6.

Swinton, J., & Pattison, S. (2010). Moving beyond clarity: Towards a thin, vague, and useful understanding of spirituality in nursing care. *Nursing Philosophy*, *11*(4), 226–237.

US Centers for Disease Control and Prevention. (2016). Alzheimer's disease: Promoting health and independence for an aging population: At a glance 2016. Retrieved October 27, 2016, from www.cdc.gov/chronicdisease/resources/publications/aag/alzheimers.htm

van der Lee, J., Bakker, J., Duivenvoorden, H. & Dröes, A-M. (2017). Do determinants of burden and emotional distress in dementia caregivers change over time? *Aging & Mental Health 21*(3), 232–240.

van Gennip, I. E., Pasman, H. R. W., Oosterveld-Vlug, M. G., Willems, D. L., & Onwuteaka-Philipsen, B. D. (2014). How dementia affects personal dignity: A qualitative study on the perspective of individuals with mild to moderate dementia. *The Journals of Gerontology Series B: Psychological Sciences and Social Sciences, 71*(3), 491–501.

Weaks, D., Wilkinson, H., & McLeod, J. (2015). Daring to tell: The importance of telling others about a diagnosis of dementia. *Ageing and Society, 35*(4), 765–784.

Wiersma, E. C., O'Connor, D. L., Loiselle, L., Hickman, K., Heibein, B., Hounam, B., & Mann, J. (2016). Creating space for citizenship: The impact of group structure on validating the voices of people with dementia. *Dementia, 15*(3), 414–433.

Wimo, A., & Prince, M. (2010). *World Alzheimer report 2010*. London, England: Alzheimer's Disease International. Retrieved from www.alz.co.uk/research/files/WorldAlzheimerReport2010.pdf

Winblad, B., Amouyel, P., Andrieu, S., Ballard, C., Brayne, C., Brodaty, H., . . . Fratiglioni, L. (2016). Defeating Alzheimer's disease and other dementias: A priority for European science and society. *The Lancet Neurology, 15*(5), 455–532.

World Health Organization. (1992). *The ICD-10 classification of mental and behavioural disorders: Clinical descriptions and diagnostic guidelines*. Geneva, Switzerland: Author. Retrieved from http://apps.who.int/iris/handle/10665/37958

World Health Organization. (2016). Dementia fact sheet. Retrieved July 29, 2016, from www.who.int/mediacentre/factsheets/fs362/en/

Wright, R. S., Waldstein, S. R., Kuczmarski, M. F., Pohlig, R. T., Gerassimakis, C. S., Gaynor, B., . . . Zonderman, A. (2016). Diet quality and cognitive function in an urban sample: Findings from the Healthy Aging in Neighborhoods of Diversity across the Life Span (HANDLS) study. *Public Health Nutrition, 2016*, 92–101. DOI:10.1017/S1368980016001361

Xiao, L. D., Wang, J., He, G.-P., De Bellis, A., Verbeeck, J., & Kyriazopoulos, H. (2014). Family caregiver challenges in dementia care in Australia and China: A critical perspective. *BMC Geriatrics, 14*(6). Retrieved from www.biomedcentral.com/1471-2318/14/6

Zelig, H. (2014). Dementia as a cultural metaphor. *The Gerontologist, 54*(2), 258–267.

Websites listed in text

Dementia Alliance International (DAI): www.dementiaallianceinternational.org/

European Working Group of People with Dementia: www.alzheimer-europe.org/Alzheimer-Europe/Who-we-are/European-Working-Group-of-People-with-Dementia

Muistiliitto: www.muistiliitto.fi/fi/etusivu/ (Accessed 14 January, 2017)

10 Family and generations

Key themes

- Families as a narrative container for emotion and care
- Generation includes historical position and personal lifecourse as well as family lineage
- Intergenerational relations may give rise to solidarity, conflict and ambivalence
- Services support rather than erode intergenerational family bonds
- Family associated with perpetuated inequalities and elder abuse
- Families can include both positive intergenerational discontinuity and positive othering

Intergenerational relations and families

When it comes to ageing, intergenerational relations have mostly been written about as if they existed principally in families. The family often acts as a container for emotional and caring issues in public discussion, which not only includes solidarity and support within families but also elder abuse, conflict, intergenerational competition and transmitting inequality. This collection of issues lends considerable ambiguity to the role of intergenerational relationships in policy and practice, particularly when background policy issues are in flux. Not only does the family raise strong personal feelings, it has also provoked conceptual disagreement within gerontology itself. Both trends tend to reinforce the boundaries separating family and generation from wider social issues. However, to begin to interpret these debates, family needs to be placed in a wider context to see how broader intergenerational narratives condition interactions within it.

Arber and Attias-Donfut (2000) observed that a feeling of generational belonging is created not just in the vertical dimension of family but also in the horizontal dimension of cohort. To this can be added generation in the sense of what point one has reached in the personal lifecourse. Family, here, refers to one's position in terms of lineage, the roles and expectations associated with a particular age position in relation to other family members. Cohort refers to the significance that is culturally ascribed to a group that is growing older together, its collective experience of history. Lifecourse refers to one's current position on a culturally expected or developmental life span and the existential priorities associated with the point that one has reached. This meeting point of lineage, cohort and lifecourse creates a three-dimensional space in which intuitive experience exists. As such,

> generation is experienced as a holistic combination of influences which give it its individual phenomenological flavour. . . . An individual may be in midlife in lifecourse terms but in family terms be part of a sandwiched generation and a member of the babyboomer (or Generation X) cohort. She or he may be changing from looking back to reference points in childhood, to looking forward to the amount of lifetime they might have left, wondering how competing family demands will allow them to use this time, how they can identify with younger rather than older generations, and how best to strive for self-actualisation. Their awareness of self and others is generationally inflected and an amalgam of influences which have yet to be designated or understood.
> (Biggs, Haapala & Lowenstein, 2011: 1112)

How family and generation are positioned will inform the nature of intergenerational relations, including family relationships, the politics of intergenerational resourcing (particularly in terms of social welfare) and even such matters as work-life balance and community environments.

Starting with family

Families are among the most enduring and widespread of systems and exist in nuclear or extended forms in all societies, as a means of regulating reproduction and support across generations. Furstenberg et al. (2015) suggest that 'the survival of family systems stems from their remarkable ability to transform their structure and practices in response to new demographic, social, and economic conditions' (2015: 31). As Lüscher and Hoff (2013) point out, families attract both positive and negative sentiments, and relations within them are subject to continual adjustment to external and internal sources of stress, in order to maintain their equilibrium. They arise in increasing variety, taking into account *sexual* orientation, step- or blended families, families of choice, as well as different cultural forms. They emerge as critical mediators between developing individuals and changing societies. Family is also used as a metaphor. Other forms of social organisation, such as care homes, hospitals, schools or whole areas of social policy can be considered family-like or not. Families exist both in private and in public, with systems of care often needing to negotiate the boundary between the two. The degree to which the private worlds of families become the concern of public issues is both a driver for new policy initiatives and for the classification and evaluation of family forms.

While the family is located at the meeting point of public and private spheres, it also acts as a container for certain social phenomena. In terms of continuity and discontinuity, it works principally at the level of the intergenerational – how generations pass or fail to pass things forward from one age group to the next.

This function is reflected in foundational concepts such as Erikson, Erikson and Kivnick's (1986) age stage based on generativity as identified with the creative process of child-rearing, Mannheim's (1928/1952) understanding of cultural change and development through generational succession, and Bengtson's (2001) work on solidarity within families (see Biggs, 2007, for a review). It has also come, particularly within gerontological thinking, to represent the site on which emotions and care are primarily discussed. With respect to the emotions, debate on the family perhaps sets a boundary around emotionality to prevent disruption or leakage into other areas of discourse, although as has been seen in discussion of emotional labour, this barrier is by no means water-tight. Care, on the other hand, sits squarely on the boundary between private and public responsibilities, with the holders of different ideological positions attempting to push those concerns into individual or collective space. Care is also, as Bauman (1995) reminds us, a concept where boundaries and commitments are left open ended both in terms of time and resources. The degree to which care is seen as a principal responsibility of family members or of the state forms one of the defining narratives underpinning the relationship between ageing and intergenerational relations.

Living a long life has had a number of effects on family relations. The internal structure of family, in terms of the number of years children can now share with their parents, has substantially increased the possibilities for intergenerational contact. Silverstein and Giarrusso (2013) point out that in 1900, only 50% of Americans had grandparents, whereas by 2000, it had risen to 90%. Bengtson and Lowenstein (2003) have referred to an emerging 'beanpole effect', with relatives spread generationally through time, in contrast to a traditional extended form with many relatives existing within a limited number of generational groups. Also, depending upon the timing of generations, the ages at which grandparents and parents bear their offspring, a grandparent and grandchild may differ in age by as little as 30 years or as many as 90 years (Mare, 2014). One result of these demographic changes is that at any given time, we may be able to live with and meet more age-others than in previous historical periods. And although opportunities for face-to-face interaction may have reduced through the forces of geographic dispersion and global migration, relatively rapid transportation and communication technologies create the potential for maintaining emotional ties in what Silverstein, Gans and Yang (2006) have called 'modified-extended families', ones that are geographically mobile yet emotionally close. The challenge, from an intergenerational point of view, is to establish adaptive ways for age groups to engage with each other within families and also in neighbourhoods and wider communities (Kaplan, Sanchez & Hoffman, 2017).

Changing approaches to family relationships

The way that the family and ageing have been studied is suffused with accommodations between the public and the private. Historically, it has shifted for a preoccupation with typologies to processes including multiplicity and interconnection with social systems.

At first, researchers focussed on different forms of relationship within families, in an attempt to classify interaction and form distinctive typologies. The purpose of these typologies, often tacitly rather than explicitly stated, was to identify types that functioned positively and types that did not. Functioning well was closely associated with harmonious relations that could ultimately sustain informal care. Bengtson and colleagues' (see Silverstein & Giarrusso, 2013) exploration of family solidarity was a key development in this area, both in identifying different types and in provoking counterarguments and debate. Using data from the Longitudinal Study of Generations of more than 300 four-generation families who in 1971 lived in Southern California, Roberts, Richards and Bengtson (1991) identified six forms of solidarity including associational solidarity (patterns of interaction), affectual solidarity (emotional closeness), consensual solidarity (agreement on attitudes and values), functional solidarity (exchange of material, instrumental and social support), normative solidarity (strength of commitment to familial roles) and structural solidarity (opportunity for interaction based mostly on geographic proximity). From this emerged four different relationship types: *harmonious* or *tight-knit*; *affective* or *intimate-but-distant*; *discordant* or *detached*; and *obligatory*, with a fifth relationship added to cover *sociable* versus *ambivalent*, in an attempt to include conflict-based relationships (Katz & Lowenstein, 2010).

The strength of the solidarity approach lies in its consideration of emotional bonds between generations, both as a conceptual model and a measurement tool. However, it has been criticised for overemphasising the positive attributes of family relations (Marshall, 2007) and of championing an ideology of familism (Lüscher & Pillemer, 1998). Indeed, Bengtson and Putney (2006) have explicitly connected family solidarity with social policy, claiming that it can have

> a profound but unrecognised influence on relations between age-groups at the societal level . . . the essence of multigenerational families is interdependence between generations and its members, and this will tend to mitigate schisms between age groups over scarce government resources.
>
> (2006: 28)

The underlying priority of solidarity research reflects the positioning of the relationship between ageing and the family as a social concern, with the family identified as the most significant social mechanism mediating care relations. And while it is possible to see this trend as originating from a perceived social problem, the creation of typologies was conceptualised as being very much a 'within family' affair. The core question has been 'what makes families work well', which then affects wider aspects of policy.

However, an approach that prioritises solidarity tacitly accepts the possibility that all may not be well below the surface. Indeed, much of the literature arising from psychoanalysis and from sociology positions the family negatively, as a source of conflict, rivalry and dispute (Turner, 1998; Biggs, 1999). Within the sociological tradition, generational change has been identified with cohort succession as each new generation sifts through what it finds and 'teaches us both to forget that which is no longer useful and to covet that which has yet to be won' (Mannheim, 1928/1952: 294). For the young, then, the preceding generation can mark a place to escape from. This does not fit well with reports of older adults' desire for family connection (Katz et al., 2015). It is also unclear how far a focus on youthful perspectives underlies such approaches, reflecting perhaps a form of age imperialism, a logic that is relevant during the first half of life and amplified by contemporary generational culture but fails to take intergenerational connection into account (Biggs, 2004).

Disquiet about an approach that prioritised solidarity, plus a competing focus on generational conflict, led to a renewed interest in ambivalence occurring both within families and between them and other social phenomena (Connidis, 2015). Here, questions of how generations negotiate situations that are inherently ambivalent, the degree to which families and intergenerational relationships are resilient to external pressures and the role of interdependent relationships have grown in importance.

According to Pillemer et al. (2007), ambivalence concerns 'the simultaneous existence of positive and negative sentiments in the older parent–adult child relationship' and what Connidis and McMullin (2002) describe as 'how social structural forces create contradictions and conflicts that are made manifest in the social interactions of family life and must be worked out in family members' (140). These two forms – psychological ambivalence, the relative ability to contain the simultaneous experience of positive and negative thoughts and emotions, and the impact of structural contradictions that result in contradictory expectations on conduct – generate psychosocial tensions expressed as mixed feelings. Lüscher et al. (2015) claim that intergenerational ambivalence can lead to oscillation between social and personal contradictions which may either lead to creativity or paralysis. Even when social expectations regarding family relationships seem clear, ambivalence can appear in the space between the actions people 'would like to take and what they are able to do as part of a larger whole' (Carolan, 2010). Ambivalence acknowledges a continuing tension, placing interaction 'within and between the public and private spheres' and encourages 'a mature step towards acknowledging a more complex world of multiple perspectives and emotional resilience' (Biggs, 2007: 706).

Workers in this area have generally eschewed typologies in favour of examining systems and processes. However, Lüscher and Hoff (2013), in taking us beyond the binary antagonisms of solidarity versus conflict, suggest four ways in which psychological and structural dimensions are experienced: through *solidarity*, where family members conceal 'ambivalence by stressing common feelings, orientations and goals of belonging and togetherness' (2013: 43); *captivation* where 'a continuous struggle over ambivalence' (44) exists and relationships become stressed; and *atomisation*, in which actors separate through conflict. Finally *emancipation* marks an openness to 'new forms of common action' (44) as ambivalence is recognised and acknowledged.

The relationship between ambivalence and social policy is, unsurprisingly, ambiguous. While Threadgold (2012) argued, "*Ideally* ambivalence can foster a scepticism that can be harnessed as a resource for change" (26), Hogerbrugge and

Silverstein (2015), somewhat acerbically, point out, from a solidarity position, that as 'ambivalence induces stress, reduces well-being, and, as a set of contradictory elements, is inherently unsustainable in the long term, we expect family members to attempt to negotiate, manage, and diminish the ambivalence they experience in relationships' (483). Lorenz-Meyer (2001: 18) notes that it can be unevenly distributed, identifying a

> politics of ambivalence, that is, the processes by which certain social positions are structurally spared high degrees of ambivalence or allow for an integration of opposed courses of action more easily at the expense of other positions. Individual and institutional responses have to be analysed in their enabling and constraining aspects.

According to this view, the distribution of ambivalence creates a form of social inequality, depending on the resources one has available to reduce the effects of stress, conflict and disadvantage on family life. The strength of the ambivalence approach lies in an acknowledgement of the dynamic transformations intergenerational relations can take over time and in different circumstances and in connecting broader structural dynamics to personal experience.

A consequence of these debates has been an increased awareness of the complexity of relations, both within families, between generations and in connection to wider social processes. Early work on what have been called 'linked lives' (Hagestad, 2003) had been undertaken by Elder (1985, 1998). Using the Oakland Growth Study, begun in 1920, Elder was able to track changes in people's lives as they encountered significant social change. He found that the timing of major social events interacted significantly with an individual's lifecourse position. Factors such as birth order, age and gender affected future life changes, depending upon when the events took place. Children were affected by the degree of responsibility they were expected to take within their families and how their same-gender parent was affected. A network of shared relationships meant that 'each generation is bound to the fateful decisions and events in the other's Life course' (Elder, 1985: 40).

Longitudinal studies of life chances following the Great Depression, the Second World War and the economic downturn in the 1980s in the American Midwest showed how linked individual lifetimes, family time and historical time interconnected. Whether one was a younger or older war recruit determined if events occurred advantageously or at 'untimely points' for future prospects, and whether one was at the crest of a wave or always challenged by younger cohorts determined long-term disadvantage. In a scenario reminiscent of recent recessional trends, for example, individuals who were born

> before 1911 ended up with college degrees and no place to go in the stagnant economy of the 1930s. Their alternative in many cases was to stay in school, piling up degrees. Indeed, they ended up better educated than the younger men, but aspirations had little to do with their achievement.
>
> (1998: 6)

Elder, Wu and Yuan (1993) found similar effects on generations of young Chinese who experienced the Cultural Revolution, where cohorts in a "sent-down generation" were subsequently disadvantaged in education, work careers, mate selection and family formation. The work of Elder and of Attias-Donfut and Wolff (2005) in France, demonstrated that the protective role of the family can be uneven and equivocal and can only be understood in close relationship to an individual's life stage and to cohort histories.

Arguably, renewed experience of recession and increasing inequality has highlighted the complexity of family relations and their interaction with the outside world. The focus here has been to acknowledge multiple factors shaping the forms families and interconnecting generations take with changing social circumstances. Outlining the importance of a multicausal approach, Hogerbrugge and Silverstein (2015) have focussed on methodological innovation and the importance of transitions in relationships. They found that transitions can affect intergenerational attitudes in a number of directions and include factors such as changes in employment status, degree of warmth and affection, presence of grandchildren, economic dependence and health. Mare (2014) has identified a number of interconnecting factors that affect the multigenerational transmission of inequality. These include an ability to transfer accumulated wealth, vulnerability to wider socioeconomic change, multiple forms that families can take and the effects of length of life and changing norms that influence the perceived importance of family bonds. He argues that wealth and income have stronger effects at the extreme top and bottom of societies. It should not be forgotten here that families are one of the main mechanisms for transmitting inequality and perpetuating cumulative disadvantage (Lorenz-Meyer, 2001; Dannefer & Kelley-Moore, 2008; Brannen, 2014). Speaking from the United Kingdom, Brannen states that 'inequalities come about for those at the bottom of the wealth and income pyramid since there is little trickle-down effect from older to younger generations. By contrast at the top of the income and wealth pyramid, assets cascade down the generational hierarchy' (2014: 486).

Taken together, such points indicate that a tendency to concentrate on typologies may be little help if these are seen as simply addressing behaviours within families. And it is here that longitudinal studies, studies of psychosocial ambivalence and of inequality show their value. A multilevel treatment of intergenerational relations is therefore key in addressing how what happens inside families connects with what happens outside them. These tensions give rise to a number of issues being identified as social problems.

Family, generation and social problems

Elder mistreatment

Discourses on family caring appear split between calls for greater support for informal carers without whom services would collapse (Winblad et al., 2016) and the demonising of carers as potential abusers. Prevalence data on elder mistreatment (abuse plus neglect) are now available from several locations: UK (2.6–3.8%:

2007), Spain (0.8–4.0%: 2007), Ireland (2.2%: 2011), New York (7.6%: 2011) and Canada (7.5–8.2%: 2016) (Tinker, Biggs, & Manthorpe, 2017). Prevalence is important because the sample population has been randomly selected, and once you have a figure, you can apply it to any population or area and get an estimate of those at risk. Prevalence can be contrasted to incidence, which tells you how many people are being picked up by services.

Figures from the UK prevalence study of elder mistreatment (Biggs et al., 2009a) indicate that 51% of mistreatment had been carried out by a partner or spouse, 49% by another family member, 13% by a care worker and 5% by a close friend. These patterns varied with type of mistreatment. Neglect was mostly by partners (70%). Partners (57%) and other family members (37%) were the main perpetrators of interpersonal (physical or psychological) abuse. A different pattern was observed for financial abuse, where the main perpetrators were family members other than spouses (54%) and care workers (31%), compared to only 13% for partners. Men were predominantly the perpetrators of interpersonal abuse (80%), whereas the gender split for financial abuse was more equal (56% men, 44% women). The age profile of perpetrators tended to be younger for those carrying out financial abuse than for those carrying out interpersonal abuse. These figures are typical of the profile found in other prevalence studies and would lead one to believe that abuse is a family affair.

However, there are problems with such conclusions. First, both the WHO (2002) and the US National Research Council's (Bonnie & Wallace, 2003) definitions, which have guided most studies, restrict abuse to the interpersonal – 'relationships of trust' or 'caregiver' – so that wider forms of mistreatment would not be counted. By contrast, the UK study also identified neighbourhood abuse as an additional form, while a study by Hong Kong Christian Services (Yan & Tang, 2004) identified community or social abuse where victims are systematically excluded from family or community participation. An article in the *British Medical Journal* (Mysyuk et al., 2015) identified 'social abuse', including systemic and institutional processes, thus more closely aligning mistreatment with ageism. Second, all prevalence studies to date have been restricted to self-reports of people living in community settings, thus excluding people living in residential care or with dementia. A report for the UK Department of Health indicated that methodological problems, such as access to a random sample of respondents, made figures for residential or hospital care impossible beyond measures of incidence (Biggs et al., 2009b). That abuse may be as much intergenerational as spousal is indicated by a number of reports. The Australian Institute of Family Studies report (Kaspiew, Carson & Rhoades, 2016) found that we need greater 'understanding of the social dynamics that may influence elder abuse, including intergenerational wealth transfer and the systemic structures that intersect with elder abuse' (16). A model based on intergenerational mediation was recommended. Finally, the Canadian Prevalence Study (MacDonald, 2016) identified 'a new and significant predictor of elder mistreatment, with abuse at earlier stages in life (childhood, youth and middle age) significantly correlated with elder abuse in later life' (3). When the limitations of current evidence are taken into account, it would appear unwise to overassociate abuse with families, per se. Indeed, in an early paper, Biggs (1996) noted a change in direction from government inquiries into institutional mistreatment to family forms that accompanied the privatisation of UK residential-care services. Since that date, a number of the countries that have undertaken prevalence studies – the United Kingdom, Ireland, Holland, the United States and Canada – have experienced an erosion of state services with families being expected to pick up the costs of care. Traditional values of inheritance and transmission thereby come into direct conflict with social policy, influencing whether assets are viewed as individual or family resources. When abuse is placed in the context of changing policies, social ageism and rights approaches, it may be wiser to interrogate the social processes that make it more or less visible than to limit it exclusively to interpersonal issues (Biggs & Haapala, 2013).

Exchanges and transfers between generations

The general aim of family policy has been to support the nuclear family in child-rearing, as a means of ensuring a stable current and future working population. Only recently have calls for support for care of people with disabilities and older adults been made (Biggs & Carr, 2015). The nuclear family is relatively disconnected from neighbourhood and intergenerational ties; it is small sized, independent, relatively mobile and tailored to the needs of production (Parsons & Bales, 1955).

A number of writers have argued that such independence may be an inappropriate goal in old age (Plath, 2008; Grenier & Phillipson, 2014; Johnston, Bailey & Wilson, 2014), where interdependence and attachment to neighbourhood may better fit older adults' lifecourse priorities. Neighbourhood appears important across cultures (Chan & Cao, 2015; Lindenberg & Westendorp, 2015; Brasher & Winterton, 2015; Moulaert & Garon, 2015), and as people grow older, their homes and the quality of the immediate neighbourhood become increasingly important as a determinant of life quality (Scharf, Phillipson & Smith, 2005).

Independence has nevertheless become the gold standard by which daily living and social inclusion are assessed (Plath, 2008; Silverstein, Conroy & Gans, 2012). Plath (2008) has suggested that this is inappropriate in so far as it places priorities from younger phases of the lifecourse onto old age that may no longer be appropriate. It creates, she argues, misunderstandings between elders, adult children and caring professionals if 'getting back to independence' is an unrealistic goal, which can cause anxiety and depression. Generating multigenerational resilience in later life may depend upon communicating humour, coping under stress and maintaining participation, mobility and security (Johnston et al., 2014). Here, maintaining intergenerational engagement may depend upon the right combination of self-protection and connection to others, rather than a concentration on independence per se (Biggs & Lowenstein, 2011). As Johnston et al. (2014) point out, 'Within multigenerational interdependence, family members recognize that their paradigm and related rules will and should shift with time. Further, they are able to adapt to such changes and continue to remain connected despite changes' (Johnston et al., 2014: 156).

Calls for independence, both personal and familial, are therefore as likely to emerge from the priorities of other age groups and the demands of macroeconomic flexibility as they are from older adults' life circumstances. And this combination is reflected in the dominant discourse on intergenerational family connection, mediated through the medium of material transfers and exchange. How, in other words, should families take care of themselves as closed systems, independent of the state.

Katz et al. (2015) found that in Europe and Israel, the most common exchange pattern was "downward familialism" in which support flowed from older parents to adult children. "Ascending familialism" was associated with a higher age of parents, health problems and higher levels of resources among adult children. These patterns were true of two-thirds of families, while others gave minimal support. Because a guaranteed transfer of support in old age is uncertain, Silverstein et al. (2012) refer to the importance of moral capital within American families and review a number of strategies that might be used by elders to ensure familial support. These include: modelling positive behaviour towards older relatives when their children are young, emulating positive intergenerational patterns in families where they exist, altruism or reliance on spiritual or religious codes and coercion through the contingent promise of inheritance. Achieving some form of equity in exchange is the desired goal, where financial support to adult children might be reciprocated by functional, everyday support as one reaches old age. As immediate reciprocity may be more difficult in old age, a longitudinal perspective may be called for, in what Antonucci (2001) has referred to as a 'support bank'. Here, earlier investments in other generations can be drawn down on in later, more vulnerable years. One of the most commonly researched questions is whether adult children who receive benefits are the same people who give support, to which Silverstein et al. (2012) and French researchers Jellal and Wolff (2007) report positively. If parents give in midlife, they are likely to receive support from the beneficiaries in old age. They argue that such strengthened solidarity results from a combination of altruism and self-interest in moral capital over time, so that even when relations are strained in later years, reciprocity is maintained.

Johnston et al. (2014) argue that exchange models imported from economics do not work well to explain family behaviour because they are overly concerned with the achievement of instrumental goals, are not contained by complex networks of emotional expectations and histories and assume equal power between parties. As Biggs and Powell (2001) have observed, market models assume a free exchange between independent parties who both then return to their own private activities and these rules rarely correspond to care or family and community bonds. Indeed, many of the assumptions held in the public domain about intergenerational relations, that older adults are perceived to be a burden and that younger people resent and eschew contact, are not supported by research. A number of studies indicate that younger adults do not resent caring for older relatives, rather, they want the right work-life balance that allows it (Gentrans, 2005–2009; Gallup Singapore, 2011; Daatland, Veenstra & Herlofson, 2012; Biggs et al., 2017). Neither may younger adults resent paying for others' pensions and health; they just want the same commitment for themselves when their time comes (Arza & Kohli, 2008;

Keck & Blome, 2008; Komp & van Tilburg, 2010). These raise a very different set of policy questions to those traditionally associated with intergenerational relations. Indeed, Boersch-Supan, Heller and Reil-Held (2011) found little evidence of a gerontocratic and self-interested voting bloc, when using data from the European SHARE survey. They reported greater trust between generations and fewer experiences of age discrimination in EU countries with larger older populations and 'no evidence that the burden of population ageing, measured by the old age dependency ration, is systematically related to a broad array of indicators for generational conflict' (2011: 20).

Intergenerational attitudes, welfare and rivalry politics

Nevertheless, a combination of population ageing and perceived fiscal threats has tied debate over exchanges between generations to a further roll back of welfare services. The ideology of non-intervention to support families arises from the belief that public and private responsibilities exist in separate spheres and that public intervention contaminates the propensity for families to look after their own if left alone to do it (Litwak, 1985). Services and state support therefore 'crowd out' natural caring and add a fiscal burden to those unaffected or able to fund support from private means. Collective responsibility for older persons and their past contribution is seen as corrosive of family responsibility. Counter to this argument, and based on a study of decision making in UK families, Finch (1995) has noted that ideologies of obligation are unsuited to contemporary family care based on affection. Further, there is no guarantee that families can take up this slack. Furstenberg et al.'s (2015) MacArthur Foundation review for the US government concludes,

> As the pressure mounts to reduce the public costs of supporting rapidly aging societies, responsibility for supporting elderly people will increasingly fall on their family members. . . . The pressures on an already overburdened and rapidly changing family system suggest that we could begin to see a diminution (if not a full reversal) of the downward flows of assistance from elderly parents and relatives to younger generations.
>
> (Furstenberg et al., 2015: 38)

They argue that the most hard hit will be middle-income families who are too rich to receive benefits yet not rich enough to balance the multiple demands of children and parents. In this context, Silverstein et al. (2012) propose that state support for its older citizens embodies a 'collective form of moral capital that, similar to its family-based counterpart, has compulsory elements (through taxation) and is reproduced across generations as a socially desirable end (manifest through stability in the political structure)' (1258).

Evidence tends to support the value of state support (Motel-Klingebiel, Tesch-Roemer & Von Kondratowitz, 2005). In Europe, while the emphasis given to family or state-based care varies from northern to southern countries (Lowenstein &

Daatland, 2006) and from east to west (Daatland, Herlofson & Lima, 2011), there is little evidence that state services negatively affect family relations. Rather, the provision of services tends to allow older and younger relatives to share more interests and activities, unencumbered by the tasks of physical tending. Thus, 'where the welfare state is more developed, it has moderated the demanding character of family obligations and allowed a more independent relationship between the generations to form' (2011: 1159). 'Where welfare benefits are universal and defined as individual rights, they allow more autonomy between generations' (Daatland et al., 2012: 134). Intergenerational bonds showed little variation from one regime to another. Services can influence the quality of relationships but do not appear to erode them.

In situations where changes in policy contradict lifetime expectations, a number of studies chart the disillusion and sense of betrayal that families feel when state support is withdrawn. From the UK, Hillcoat-Nallétamby and Phillips (2011) report negative ambivalence being exacerbated by shortages in public alternatives to family care. Dutch authors present a 'narrative of loss in which the state formerly reduced the pressure on families by supporting older adults but now is retreating from a social welfare approach' (Van den Broek, Dykstra & Romke, 2015: 261). By contrast, where state support has been increased, as in some emerging economies, intergenerational reciprocity provides benefits: 'The introduction of old-age pensions – frequently the first step of public social assistance, greatly improves the financial position of the elderly and may lead to a reversal of the financial flow by enabling them to aid the families of their adult children and help cover the schooling expenses of their grandchildren' (United Nations Department of Economic and Social Affairs, 2004: 4.2 33).

This view is supported by evidence by Aboderin and Hoffman's (2015) report on West Africa. While the effects of rapid social change in China has increased demands for state support for older adults (Du & Xie, 2015), early attempts, in 2013, to simply enforce filial responsibility were quickly withdrawn.

Daatland et al.'s (2012) Norwegian study found that intergenerational attitudes were balanced towards altruism in the family and towards self-interest regarding the welfare state. They also found that lifecourse position influenced perceived need, such that people became aware of issues as they approach certain phases of life, such as one's own parents ageing and eventually one's own old age. While midlifers had low expectations of intergenerational support, women were the most in favour of state intervention. There was again little evidence of generational conflict. Indeed, Attias-Donfut and Wolff (2005) draw attention to the power of oral history passed on through families as a means of resistance to official versions of events.

A Pew Research Center (2015) study of the United States, Germany and Italy found widespread concerns about the future of social security, but 'compared with Americans, twice as many Germans and even more Italians think the government should bear greatest responsibility for people's economic wellbeing in their old age'. Marcum and Treas (2013) surveyed evidence from 27 countries and found that while interest in favour of one's own group predominated in the United States,

European interests tended to reflect general attitudes to state support independent of generational position. Intergenerational contracts were weakest in liberal economies and highest in social-democratic, postsocialist and conservative regimes. In all cases, societies with a tradition of female employment were more supportive of welfare. They conclude that 'there may be a greater receptivity to a focus on functional solidarity that emphasises needs of and obligations throughout the lifecourse, rather than singling out any particular age group . . . and . . . there is no evidence of much support for a retreat from the welfare state' (2013: 307).

In spite of this evidence, a number of agencies have attempted to stoke intergenerational rivalry. Generational rivalry first appeared as a policy issue in the United States in the Reaganite 1980s as a debate over 'generational equity' aimed to reduce payments to the old (Williamson, McNamara & Howling, 2003), also referred to as the 'age-race wars' (Minkler & Robertson, 1991). Here, the aim was to divide interest groups to facilitate general cuts to public support. It has, in the 21st century, been revived to account for housing shortages, casualised work and a low-wage economy facing younger adults. While the evidence is reasonably clear that the advantages experienced by the previous generation are not causally related to the disadvantages faced by their children, this does not stop the debate being posed in the media as one of generational conflict (see for example BBC 2017: www.bbc.com/news/business-38558116) as marginal political debates elbow their way into the mainstream. The Grattan Institute (Dailey & Wood, 2014) in Australia and the Intergenerational Foundation (2015) in the United Kingdom have both lobbied government to reduce the benefits given to older generations to pay for the needs of other age groups. Both reports cite the rising costs of housing, education and low wages as serious problems facing people in their twenties and thirties. In both cases, that lifetime income will not rise so quickly for younger generations, though projected to be higher relative to older generations, was seen to require a programme of 'intergenerational rebalancing'. This consisted in reducing support to older adults, rather than re-introducing the policies that had supported the boomer generation. In the context of cultural disquiet about the general distribution of wealth, associating economic inequality with generational inequity has returned as a political option. In fact, since Piketty (2014), it is commonly accepted that social inequality has risen significantly and that the extreme difference between the poor and rich of all generations creates a brake on economic progress.

While the politics of generational rivalry recognises generational difference, it has become stuck in antagonism without rising to discover an encompassing intergenerational solution. Rather than attempting to resolve ambivalence, it opts for conflict. In this sense, it would be an example of simple rather than complex generational thinking, what Biggs and Lowenstein (2011) identify as low generational intelligence – thinking that cannot take the position of the other into account. And while with a bit of luck, we will each move into the place of the age-other over time, this approach appears stuck in a form of present-centredness, which attempts to block considering how the advantages of previous generations may be re-built and regained from a longitudinal and lifecourse perspective. When looked at from a lifetime-centred approach, competition between generations is essentially fruitless at a macrotemporal level, as one is eventually competing against one's own future.

In a different voice, Generations United USA claim that "public policy should meet the needs of all generations. . . . Resources are more wisely used when they connect generations rather than separate them" (2017, January 14). Like Biggs and Lowenstein (2011) and Kaplan et al. (2017) recommend, the development of intergenerational negotiation of 'meta-generational policies' is proposed 'taking into account individual generations, looking, above all, to the relationships between all generations and not just to each generation on its own' (137). Each are in sympathy with the United Nations Millennium Development Goals (2007) that 'governments are considering instruments that can improve the well-being of young and older generations rather than focusing on one particular group' and that 'Though intergenerational solidarity may appear natural and result from altruism and good will, bonds between different generations must be created and promoted intentionally' (United Nations, 2007: 10).

Each of these approaches holds the promise of increasing positive othering based on complementary intergenerational relations and a move from present to lifetime-centred thinking.

Concluding comments

The landscape on which ageing, family and intergenerational relations intersect is increasingly becoming contested. The family has been seen as a container for emotions and attitudes to care, protecting other areas of gerontological debate from potentially explosive and divisive issues. And while attempts have been made to emphasise the power of generational solidarity, this would rely upon finding a means of negotiating the often ambivalent feelings and beliefs that intergenerational relations can provoke. These relations have themselves been turned into problems mediated by the language of exchange and transfers of resources as part of a wider debate on who should care for the most old. In the public sphere, debates have been revived over generational rivalry, even though these initiatives appear not to be supported by evidence. It is also a long way from arguing that families can support positive intergenerational relations to assuming that families can replace supportive structures that have been taken away. Both are most likely to provoke tension between generations and divert attention from more pervasive causes of social inequality.

An often-overlooked element of this debate is how generational continuity and discontinuity has been positioned, an issue that cannot be fully explained by transfers and exchanges. The main question here appears to be how to live with transitions that are also sources of sustained continuity. Families contain elements of both continuity across generations and positive discontinuity through the complementary contributions of different age groups. They also have the potential to incorporate generational distinctiveness and positive othering, which may be generalizable to comprehend other forms of intergenerational negotiation. Because intergenerational relations hold the possibility of being both present- and lifetime-centred, they also promise to span within- and between-age thinking. And it is perhaps in this sense that we can learn from them as a contribution to public debate. The ways in which wider events can influence intergenerational connections and how generations can negotiate mutually agreeable solutions are key issues in taking us forward if we are to adapt culturally.

References

Aboderin, I., & Hoffman, J. (2015). Families, intergenerational bonds, and aging in Sub-Saharan Africa. *Canadian Journal on Aging/La Revue canadienne du vieillissement, 34*(3), 282–289.

Antonucci, T. C. (2001). Social relations an examination of social networks, social support. In J. Birren & K. Schaie (Eds.), *Handbook of the psychology of aging* (pp. 427–453). New York, NY: Academic Press.

Arber, S., & Attias-Donfut, C. (2000). *The myth of generational conflict.* London, England: Routledge.

Arza, C., & Kohli, M. (2008). *Pension reform in Europe: Politics, policies and outcomes* (1st ed.). New York, NY: Routledge.

Attias-Donfut, C., & Wolff, F. C. (2005). Generational memory and family relationships. In M. L. Johnson (Ed.), *The Cambridge handbook of age and ageing* (pp. 443–454). Cambridge, England: Cambridge University Press.

Bauman, Z. (1995). *Life in fragments: Essays in postmodern morality.* Oxford, England: Blackwell.

Bengtson, V. L. (2001). The burgess award lecture: Beyond the nuclear family: The increasing importance of multigenerational bonds. *Journal of Marriage and the Family, 63*(1), 1–16.

Bengtson, V. L., & Lowenstein, A. (2003). *Global aging and challenges to families.* New York, NY: Aldine de Gruyter.

Bengtson, V. L., & Putney, N. M. (2006). Two future "conflicts" across generations and cohorts? In J. A. Vincent, C. Phillipson & M. Downs (Eds.), *The futures of old age* (pp. 20–29). London, England: Sage.

Biggs, S. (1996). A family concern: Elder abuse in British social policy. *Critical Social Policy, 16*(2), 63–88.

Biggs, S. (1999). *The mature imagination: Dynamics of identity in midlife and beyond.* Buckingham, England: Open University Press.

Biggs, S. (2004). New ageism: Age imperialism, personal experience and ageing policy. In S.-O. Daatland & S. Biggs (Eds.), *Ageing and diversity: Multiple pathways and cultural migrations* (pp. 95–106). Bristol, England: Policy Press.

Biggs, S. (2007). Thinking about generations: Conceptual positions and policy implications. *Journal of Social Issues, 63*(4), 695–712.

Biggs, S., & Carr, A. (2015). Work, aging, and risks to family life: The case of Australia. *Canadian Journal on Aging/La Revue canadienne du vieillissement, 34*(3), 321–330.

Biggs, S., & Haapala, I. (2013). Elder mistreatment, ageism, and human rights. *International Psychogeriatrics, 25*(8), 1299–1306.

Biggs, S., Haapala, I., & Lowenstein, A. (2011). Exploring generational intelligence as a model for examining the process of intergenerational relationships. *Ageing and Society, 31*(7), 1107–1124.

Biggs, S., & Lowenstein, A. (2011). *Generational intelligence: A critical approach to age relations.* New York, NY: Routledge.

Biggs, S., Manthorpe, J., McCreadie, C., Tinker, A., Doyle, M., & Erens, B. (2009a). Mistreatment of older people in the United Kingdom: Findings from the first national prevalence study. *Journal of Elder Abuse & Neglect, 21*(1), 1–14.

Biggs, S., McGann, M., Bowman, D., & Kimberley, H. (2017). Work, health and the commodification of life's time: Reframing work – life balance and the promise of a long life. *Ageing and Society, 37*(7), 1458–1483.

Biggs, S., & Powell, J. L. (2001). A Foucauldian analysis of old age and the power of social welfare. *Journal of Aging & Social Policy, 12*(2), 93–112.

Biggs, S., Stevens, M., Tinker, A., Dixon, J., & Lee, L. (2009, December). *Institutional mistreatment and dignity: Toward a conceptual understanding.* A working paper for the Department of Health and Comic Relief. Unpublished document.

Boersch-Supan, A., Heller, G., & Reil-Held, A. (2011). Is intergenerational cohesion falling apart in old Europe? *Public Policy and Aging Report, 21*(4), 17–21.

Bonnie, R. J., & Wallace, R. B. (2003). *Elder mistreatment: Abuse, neglect and exploitation in an aging America.* Washington, DC: National Research Council.

Brannen, J. (2014). From the concept of generation to an intergenerational lens on family lives. *Families, Relationships and Societies, 3*(3), 485–489.

Brasher, K., & Winterton, G. (2015). Whose responsibility? In T. Moulaert & S. Garon (Eds.), *Age-friendly cities and communities in international comparison: Political lessons, scientific avenues, and democratic issues* (pp. 229–247). New York, NY: Springer Publishing Company.

Carolan, M. (2010). Sociological ambivalence and climate change. *Local Environment, 15,* 309–321. DOI:10.1080/13549831003677662

Chan, A. C. M., & Cao, T. (2015). Age-friendly neighbourhoods as civic participation: Implementation of an active ageing policy in Hong Kong. *Journal of Social Work Practice, 29*(1), 53–68.

Connidis, I. A. (2015). Exploring ambivalence in family ties: Progress and prospects. *Journal of Marriage and Family, 77,* 77–79.

Connidis, I. A., & McMullin, J. A. (2002). Sociological ambivalence and family ties: A critical perspective. *Journal of Marriage and Family, 64,* 558–567.

Daatland, S. O., Herlofson, K., & Lima, I. A. (2011). Balancing generations: On the strength and character of family norms in the West and East of Europe. *Ageing and Society, 31*(7), 1159–1179.

Daatland, S. O., Veenstra, M., & Herlofson, K. (2012). Age and intergenerational attitudes in the family and the welfare state. *Advances in Life Course Research, 17*(3), 133–144.

Dailey, J., & Wood, D. (2014). *The wealth of generations.* Melbourne, Australia: The Grattan Institute.

Dannefer, D., & Kelley-Moore, J. (2008). New twists in the paths of the life course. In V. Bengtson, M. Silverstein & N. Putney (Eds.), *Handbook of theories of aging* (pp. 389–409). New York, NY: Springer Publishing Company.

Du, P., & Xie, L. (2015). The use of law to protect and promote age-friendly environment. *Journal of Social Work Practice, 29*(1), 13–21.

Elder, G. H., Jr. (Ed.). (1985). *Life course dynamics: Trajectories and transitions, 1968–1980.* Ithaca, NY: Cornell University Press.

Elder, G. H., Jr. (1998). The life course and human development. In R. M. Lerner (Ed.), W. Damon (General Ed.), *Handbook of child psychology, Vol. 1: Theoretical models of human development* (5th ed., pp. 939–991). New York, NY: Wiley.

Elder, G. H., Jr., Wu, W., & Yuan, J. (1993). *State-initiated change and the life course in Shanghai, China.* Unpublished project report. In Elder, G. H., Jr. (2001). Families, social change, and individual lives. *Marriage & Family Review,* 177–192.

Erikson, E. G., Erikson, J. M., & Kivnick, H. Q. (1986). *Vital involvement in old age*. New York, NY: W.W. Norton & Company.

Finch, J. (1995). Responsibilities, obligations and commitments. In I. Allen & E. Perkins (Eds.), *The future of family care for older people* (pp. 51–64). London, England: HMSO.

Furstenberg, F. F., Hartnett, C. S., Kohli, M., & Zissimopoulos, J. M. (2015). The future of intergenerational relations in aging societies. *Daedalus, 144*(2), 31–40.

Gallup Singapore. (2011). *C3A survey in intergenerational relationships and ageing*. Unpublished research report.

Gentrans. (2005–2009). "Baby boomers" generational transmissions in Finland': The GENTRANS research project. University of Helsinki and Statistics Finland. Retrieved October 11, 2016, from http://blogs.helsinki.fi/gentrans/

Grenier, A., & Phillipson, C. (2014). Rethinking agency in late life. In J. Baars, J. Dohmen, A. Grenier & C. Phillipson (Eds.), *Ageing, meaning and social structure: Connecting critical and humanistic gerontology* (pp. 55–80). Bristol, UK: Policy Press.

Hagestad, G. O. (2003). Interdependent lives and relationships in changing times: A life-course view of families and aging. In R. Settersten (Ed.), *Invitation to the life course toward new understanding of later life* (pp. 135–59). Amityville, NY: Baywood.

Hillcoat-Nallétamby, S., & Phillips, J. E. (2011). Sociological ambivalence revisited. *Sociology, 45*, 202–217.

Hogerbrugge, M. J., & Silverstein, M. D. (2015). Transitions in relationships with older parents: From middle to later years. *The Journals of Gerontology Series B: Psychological Sciences and Social Sciences, 70*(3), 481–495.

The Intergenerational Foundation. (2015). Intergenerational fairness index 2015. Retrieved December 6, 2015, from www.if.org.uk/archives/6909/2015-intergenerational-fairness-index

Jellal, M., & Wolff, F. C. (2007). Cultural evolutionary altruism: Theory and evidence. *European Journal of Political Economy, 18*, 241–262.

Johnston, J. H., Bailey, W. A., & Wilson, G. (2014). Mechanisms for fostering multigenerational resilience. *Contemporary Family Therapy, 36*(1), 148–161.

Kaplan, M., Sanchez, M., & Hoffman, J. (2017). Intergenerational approaches for sustaining individual health and well-being. In M. Kaplan, M. Sanchez & J. Hoffman (Eds.), *Intergenerational pathways to a sustainable society* (pp. 29–64). New York, NY: Springer International Publishing.

Kaspiew, R., Carson, C., & Rhoades, H. (2016). *Elder abuse understanding issues, frameworks and responses*. Research Report No. 35. AIFS: Melbourne.

Katz, R., & Lowenstein, A. (2010). Theoretical perspectives on intergenerational solidarity, conflict and ambivalence. In M. Izuhara (Ed.), *Ageing and intergenerational relations* (pp. 29–57). Bristol, UK: Policy Press.

Katz, R., Lowenstein, A., Halperin, D., & Tur-Sinai, A. (2015). Generational solidarity in Europe and Israel. *Canadian Journal on Aging/La Revue canadienne du vieillissement, 34*(3), 342–355.

Keck, W., & Blome, A. (2008). Is there a generational cleavage in Europe? In J. Alber, T. Fahey & C. Saraceno (Eds.), *Handbook of quality of life in the enlarged European Union* (1st ed., pp. 70–100). London, England: Routledge.

Komp, K., & van Tilburg, T. (2010). Ageing societies and the welfare state: Where the inter-generational contract is not breached. *International Journal of Ageing and Later Life, 5*(1), 7–11.

Lindenberg, J., & Westendorp, R. G. (2015). Overcoming old in age-friendliness. *Journal of Social Work Practice, 29*(1), 85–98.

Litwak, E. (1985). *Helping the elderly: The complementary roles of informal networks and formal systems.* New York, NY: Guilford Press.

Lorenz-Meyer, D. (2001). *The politics of ambivalence* (Gender Institute New Working Paper). Konstanz University, Germany. Series 2: 1–24.

Lowenstein, A., & Daatland, S. O. (2006). Filial norms and family support in a comparative cross-national context: Evidence from the OASIS study. *Ageing & Society, 26*(1), 1–21.

Lüscher, K., & Hoff, A. (2013). Intergenerational ambivalence: Beyond solidarity and conflict. In I. Albert & D. Ferring (Eds.), *Intergenerational relations: European perspectives on family and society* (pp. 39–63). Bristol, England: University of Bristol.

Lüscher, K., Hoff, A., Lamura, G., Renzi, M., Sánchez, M., Viry, G., & de Salles Oliveira, P. (2015). *Generations, intergenerational relationships, generational policy: A multilingual compendium.* Konstanz, Germany: Konstanz University Press.

Lüscher, K., & Pillemer, K. (1998). Intergenerational ambivalence: A new approach to the study of parent-child relations in later life. *Journal of Marriage and the Family, 60,* 413–425.

MacDonald, L. (2016). *Into the light: National survey on the mistreatment of older Canadians.* Toronto, Canada: NICE.

Mannheim, K. (1928/1952). The problem of generations. In P. Kecskemeti (Ed.), *Essays on the sociology of knowledge* (pp. 276–319). London, England: Routledge and Kegal Paul.

Marcum, C. S., & Treas, J. (2013). The intergenerational social contract revisited. In M. Silverstein & R. Giarrusso (Eds.), *Kinship and cohort in an aging society: From generation to generation* (pp. 293–313). Baltimore, MD: Johns Hopkins University Press.

Mare, R. D. (2014). Multigenerational aspects of social stratification: Issues for further research. *Research in Social Stratification and Mobility, 35,* 121–128.

Marshall, V. W. (2007). Advancing the sociology of ageism. *Social Forces, 86,* 257.

Minkler, M., & Robertson, A. (1991). The ideology of age-race wars. *Ageing and Society, 11*(1), 1–22.

Motel-Klingebiel, A., Tesch-Roemer, C., & Von Kondratowitz, H. (2005). Welfare states do not crowd out the family: Evidence for mixed responsibility from comparative analyses. *Ageing and Society, 25*(6), 863–882. DOI:10.1017/S0144686X05003971

Moulaert, T., & Garon, S. (Eds.). (2015). *Age-friendly cities and communities in international comparison: Political lessons, scientific avenues, and democratic issues.* New York, NY: Springer Publishing Company.

Mysuyk, Y., Westendorp, R. G. J., Biggs, S., & Lindenberg, J. (2015). Listening to the voices of abused older people: Should we classify system abuse? *BMJ: British Medical Journal (Online), 350,* h2697.

Parsons, T., & Bales, F. (1955). *Family, socialization and interaction process.* New York, NY: Free Press.

Pew Research Center. (2015). Americans are aging, but not as fast as people in Germany, Italy and Japan. Retrieved October 11, 2016, from www.pewresearch.org/fact-tank/2015/05/21/americans-are-aging-but-not-as-fast-as-people-in-germany-italy-and-japan/

Piketty, T. (2014). *Capital in the twenty-first century: The dynamics of inequality, wealth, and growth.* Cambridge, MA: The Belknap Press of Harvard University Press.

Pillemer, K. A., Suitor, J., Mock, S., Sabir, M., Prado, T., & Sechrist, J. (2007). Capturing the complexity of intergenerational relations: Exploring ambivalence within later-life families. *Journal of Social Issues, 63*(4), 793–808.

Plath, D. (2008). Independence in old age: The route to social exclusion? *British Journal of Social Work, 38,* 1353–1369.

Roberts, R. E. L., Richards, L. N., & Bengtson, V. L. (1991). Intergenerational solidarity in families. In S. P. Pfeifer & M. B. Sussman (Eds.), *Families: Intergenerational and generational connections* (pp. 11–46). New York, NY: Haworth Press.

Scharf, T., Phillipson, C., & Smith, A. E. (2005). Social exclusion of older people in deprived urban communities of England. *European Journal of Ageing, 2*(2), 76–87.

Silverstein, M., Conroy, S. J., & Gans, D. (2012). Beyond solidarity, reciprocity and altruism: Moral capital as a unifying concept in intergenerational support for older people. *Ageing and Society, 32*(7), 1246–1262.

Silverstein, M., Gans, D., & Yang, F. M. (2006). Intergenerational support to aging parents the role of norms and needs. *Journal of Family Issues, 27*(8), 1068–1084.

Silverstein, M., & Giarrusso, R. (2013). *Kinship and cohort in an aging society: From generation to generation.* Baltimore, MD: Johns Hopkins University Press.

Threadgold, S. (2012). "I reckon my life will be easy, but my kids will be buggered": Ambivalence in young people's positive perceptions of individual futures and their visions of environmental collapse. *Journal of Youth Studies, 15*, 17–32.

Tinker, A., Biggs, S., & Manthorpe, J. (2017). The mistreatment and neglect of frail older people. In H. M. Fillit, L. Rockwood & J. B. Young (Eds.), *Brocklehurst's textbook of geriatric medicine and gerontology* (pp. 959–972). Philadelphia, PA: Saunders (W.B.) Company Limited (Elsevier Health Sciences).

Turner, B. S. (1998). Ageing and generational conflicts. *British Journal of Sociology, 49*, 299–304.

United Nations. (2007). Millennium development goals. Retrieved from www.un.org/millenniumgoals/

United Nations Department of Economic and Social Affairs. (2004). *World youth report 2003: The global situation of young people.* New York, NY: United Nations.

van den Broek, T., Dykstra, P., & Romke, J. (2015). Care ideals in the Netherlands: Shifts between 2002 and 2011. *Canadian Journal on Aging/La Revue canadienne du vieillissement, 34*(3), 268–281.

Williamson, J. B., McNamara, T. K., & Howling, S. A. (2003). Generational equity, generational interdependence, and the framing of the debate over social security reform. *Journal of Sociology & Social Welfare, 30*(3), 3–14.

Winblad, B., Amouyel, P., Andrieu, S., Ballard, C., Brayne, C., Brodaty, H., . . . Fratiglioni, L. (2016). Defeating Alzheimer's disease and other dementias: A priority for European science and society. *The Lancet Neurology, 15*(5), 455–532.

World Health Organization. (2002). *Missing voices: Views of older persons on elder abuse.* Geneva, Switzerland: WHO.

Yan, E. C. W., & Tang, C. S. K. (2004). Elder abuse by caregivers: A study of prevalence and risk factors in Hong Kong Chinese families. *Journal of Family Violence, 19*(5), 269–277.

Website listed in text

Generations United: www.gu.org, Accessed 14/01/2017.

Conclusions

Key themes

- Distinctive lifecourse priorities provide an alternative material base for cultural adaptation
- Adaptive personal ageing requires continuity of identity and discontinuity of priority
- A series of existing narratives requires renegotiation if cultural adaptation is to take place
- Intergenerational relations should work towards complementary solutions based on positive othering
- A lifetime-centred perspective should inform public policy debate
- Within- and between-age thinking require interconnection

This book has been written in a particular period, with growing numbers of older adults relative to other generational groups and when many of the cultural certainties of preceding years appear to be in flux. Such uncertainty provokes policy makers to fall back on pre-existing narratives and underlying priorities, often in an attempt at premature closure, perhaps in order not to think too deeply about the unthought and the knowns of a historically unprecedented phenomenon. If changing lifecourse priorities were to be recognised as an alternative material base to productivism and economic instrumentalism, negotiating ageing would be both culturally and personally more challenging. Navigating these priorities would require accrued experience and a relative awareness of finitude, combined with issues of immediate importance. It may then be possible to outline the contours of what purposes the extra years of a long life might promise and what form intergenerational relations could take in order to adapt to population ageing. These are questions that are difficult to answer without placing a long life and the effects of population ageing alongside our understanding of intergenerational relations (a theme that has been taken up elsewhere in Biggs & Lowenstein, 2011). In addition, it may be possible to reflect these observations back to our social and our human condition and see them in a new light. This raises questions about the nature of a good life and a good society. Have we got our priorities straight? How should narratives of a long life interconnect personally and generationally? What would make them sustainable and negotiable?

Four narratives on adult ageing have been outlined as they arise in public debate, personal experience and the scientific literature. Each of them contributes to the task of negotiating the cultural implications of a long life and more complex inter-generational relations. They are inevitably incomplete and perhaps one area that has not been covered in detail concerns building age-friendly environments. A review of thinking in this area can be found in Moulaert and Garon's (2016) com-pendium on age-friendly cities and communities. The choice of pursuing ageing has also happened at the expense of privileging other narratives of human experi-ence, such as gender, orientation, race and cultural diversity. Each of these are widely covered elsewhere (see for example Leime et al., 2017).

Negotiating a new set of cultural priorities for population ageing raises a series of issues that go beyond labour economics and lie in the rediscovery of whole lifetime perspectives. At a personal level, this should allow us to marry continuing selves with changing priorities. It should facilitate the finding of intergenerational solutions based on complementary rather than competitive relationships.

Of the narratives covered, it may be possible to say that while work has come to colonise what is considered to be a legitimate and active later life, evidence on its effectiveness is, to say the least, equivocal. Many of the claims made for it are simply that, crafted to fit partial economic agendas from elsewhere. Work has proved to be a singularly unreliable base on which to find a purpose for longev-ity. Nevertheless many of the arguments made in its favour have migrated from the periphery to the mainstream. Spirituality alerts us to elements of the human condition that work has no answer for other than elimination, vulnerability being the foremost. Narratives of the spirit increase awareness of liminality, the sense of living in between states, which may take the form of being between the material and the divine, transitions between different states of awareness and priority, or connectivity between generations.

The body, in both its physical and mental manifestations, exists as the principal concern of health and biomedicine. A critical analysis of naturalness, disease states and therapies associated with longevity highlights aspects of hope and fear asso-ciated with adult ageing. Interactions between the helping professions and older adults are almost inevitably intergenerational, which contributes to tensions around empathic understanding, emotional labour and professional distance. The twin narra-tives of prolongivism plus its commercial arm, anti-ageing, and of the public percep-tion of dementia, create two opposing aspects of aspirational ageing, one colonising hope and the other fear. In each case, however, the experience of ageing is eclipsed through processes of avoidance or denial and through radical forms of othering. Family, once placed in the context of wider intergenerational processes, appears surprisingly adaptive as an intimation of processes for longevity and for generational negotiation. While it is fraught with emotional contradictions and harried by policy shifts, it takes a recognition of generational distinctiveness to its core and includes a lifecourse perspective. Whether these advantages can be scaled up to social policy is fraught with contradictions, however. Family forms of relation would need to be seen as a template for collective engagement and inclusion, rather than an excuse for policy substitution and an evasion of collective social responsibilities.

Each narrative throws a particular light on questions of positive and negative othering, continuity and change and within- and between-age or present- or life-time-centred thinking. Taken together, they outline the task of interconnection that faces us.

On balance, while some amount of decent, age-friendly or age-neutral working life may be a necessary component in negotiating a long life, it is certainly not sufficient. And few people would argue that good health should not be promoted across the lifecourse. But these are means and not ends in themselves. Openness to spirit and family-like relations may provide narratives that begin to answer questions of meaning if they are linked to wider forms of civic and political engagement. What emerges is that we have a rich cultural reservoir of models to age by. However, they have largely been crafted in a context with few older and many younger adults rather than an historical period where generations are similar in size. They need to be sifted through from a long-lived and intergenerational perspective if adaptation is to be achieved. Currently, we are left with an amalgam of activity that offers more of the same, vulnerability that is both in between and potentially transformative, promises that sensationalise hope or fear, yet also the possibility of collaboration and an awareness of generational coexistence. Each of these, while separated by different policy domains and mediums of expression, may connect to shed light on what we desire from a long life and what we desire it not to be.

To understand and discriminate between these alternatives, it is argued that increased awareness of lifecourse and generation presents a new material base beyond the shifting sands of economic instrumentalism. A complex of psychosocial and bodily change draws attention to the fact that the lifecourse itself contains a materiality in terms of time as well as space. As identified elsewhere (Biggs & Lowenstein, 2011), each life phase has a distinctive set of priorities due to its position in an expanded life span. Once this is recognised, it raises the point that generations differ and a single perspective cannot be assumed to be universally valid. Thus, any one position will require negotiation between it and the others. The degree to which people become aware of this and their willingness to positively encounter the age-other indicates their degree of generational intelligence. This intelligence forms the basis of intergenerational negotiation and the creation of sustainable solutions. Lifetime-centred awareness thereby determines the relevance of present-centred thinking for the ageing project. Positive otherness is valued and positive discontinuity is valorised. However, rather than forming an excuse for generational competition, elements of each narrative offer an insight into how cooperation between generations might be configured. Work offers, in its most positive incarnation, an awareness of age-neutrality in its evocation of agelessness. However, in its ruthless pursuit of productivism, this is often hidden from view. Spirit offers unity in diversity in so far as pathways are presented as universally applicable independently of age. It also, in its sensitising force, identifies that all material states are in some way in between, promising both discontinuity and transformation. The body is malleable but not infinitely so. Continuing physical and mental health are key to continued psychosocial participation but also exhibit a strong tendency towards material avoidance or a pushing away of signifiers of age. Family offers a model that is at once inviting in its awareness of generation and disturbing if it is used to eschew collective responsibility of care and the negative discontinuities of old age.

The degree to which it is possible to use this narrative raw material to fashion or prefigure new forms of ageing and generational connection is open to debate; it is also subject to powerful forces that do not necessarily share the same interests. Perhaps it is safest to say that such prefiguration should follow the path of the least unnatural and most authentic; it should recognise the characteristic features of a life lived long and the rhythms that shape generational distinctiveness and interaction. This rediscovery of the material realities of lifecourse priorities should form the foundations of any new understanding of ageing and new forms of radical critique.

The purpose of a long life, then, is to fully work through the inherent qualities of the phase of life one is in and connect this to encounters in the here and now. It takes from both the reflective self, encountered in the United Nations' Vienna (1982) statement, and the engagement of the Madrid (2002) statement outlined in the first chapter of this book. It also requires recognition that while individuals desire continuity of identity, so to be seen as the same person throughout their lives, they also need to adapt to existential challenges that require positive discontinuity in the negotiation of age-related priorities. One is not so much lost in an unending present or living in the past, as living with the past in the service of an intergenerational future. From this flows an awareness of the complementarity of specific generational priorities. Tensions between ambivalence and solidarity, employment and retirement, health and disease, each mark contradictions struggling for resolution and the birth of a new form of growing old, which can then feed back into a wider understanding of humanity and purpose.

Adaptation to generations of equal size requires negotiation rather than a willful and unthought-through imposition of one age set of priorities over another. In the current period, pointers to common directions may lie in generations' simultaneous experiencing of the erosion of current and future life chances, with each phase of the lifecourse becoming more precarious for the majority of us. If uncertainty in everyday life is marked by income insecurity, fragmentation of identity and lack of time control, then an erosion of security in a decent job or available pension, of decent care and of a supportive state are markers that can unite the generations. In this context, within-age rather than between-age thinking plays into a scenario of division and rule. Precarity can be understood as infusing each part of the lifecourse with uncertainty and instability. The commodification of lifetime and marketisation of forms of care have certainly leached their way into the everyday lives of many older people, but when placed in a life-priorities context take on a particular character in later life in so far as finitude has become an increasing certainty while the timing and implications of such limitation are increasingly uncertain. The emotional consequences of this increased awareness provoke a particular quality of precarity, which is closely connected to the materiality of the lifecourse itself. It is not, then, simply a predicament based in work and other forms of income at particular points in the lifecourse; it also increasingly becomes a general condition of a life lived long, affecting lifetime rhythms as a whole.

So how does one negotiate a sense of authentic purpose and connection with other age groups? How does one sift through the narratives we have inherited and seek a future that sustains each generation? How do the items identified throughout this book help us as critical tools? It has perhaps been possible to discriminate between narratives in terms of positive discontinuity and positive othering, present-centred or lifetime-centred and as instances of within-age and between-age thinking. These tensions are not necessarily expressed as polar opposites, however; rather, they appear as tendencies that serve particular functions within particular narrative structures. They constellate with different force depending upon psychosocial vectors towards avoidance or denial or by embracing the complexities of ageing and of intergenerational relations. The degree to which a policy or practice concentrates on one age group or connects age groups and in what way will contribute to the way new narrative spaces are created.

Many of the narratives presented to us as ways of seeing old age reflect a desire to argue away the complex interaction of social, psychological and bodily realities of ageing and generation. Yet if we are to see clearly at all, we must overcome our desire not to experience the emotional impacts of vulnerability and ambivalence. We may then begin to assess ageing realistically rather than being anaesthetised by narrative structures that in some cases may end up to be so much wishful thinking. We need, in other words, to learn to lean selectively upon pre-existing cultural constructions while recognising that we can also influence and change them.

In terms of intergenerational sustainability, new configurations should contain the following qualities. They should last over time and therefore lend predictability; recognise the distinctive diversity of age relations, lending coherence; work towards negotiated solutions based on empathic understanding and by identifying complementary relations between age groups, support cohesion.

These novel directions should be able to embrace psychosocial discontinuities that occur as we grow and age (rather than fear or deny them), generate higher levels of generational intelligence through sustained negotiation and connect rhythms of lifecourse readiness to the processes contained in social institutions.

Does this tell us much about the human condition more generally and whether we have the right priorities? Here, we need to acknowledge that there have been attempts to separate out 'ageing' issues from intergenerational ones, compounding the disconnect between generational groups. Second, certain qualities of the human condition have been pushed into old age to minimise their effects on other phases. However, our priorities, if we are to adapt culturally, would need to return these issues so that they might re-enter our understanding of longevity and intergenerational relations. This would have a longitudinal element, in that a long life draws attention to long-term, slow-burn consequences, and a here and now element in so far as it can teach us how to build complementary relationships. The good life, then, should include an awareness of one's own life priorities, a sensitivity to those of others and spaces in which mutually enduring solutions can emerge. The creation of such spaces would be the first step of a culturally adapted social policy.

Some hints at what an approach that takes a lifetime-centred and generationally aware perspective might look like have emerged from this inquiry.

It appears, for example, when public and private perspectives are compared, that rather than seeing older adults as a burden for whom they don't want to care, younger age groups want the right work-life balance to allow them to spend more shared intergenerational time. Also, people don't mind paying for other generational groups' needs; they simply want the same deal when their time comes. Further, people want to do something distinctive, contributions that are appropriate to their current life priorities, rather than to endure a more-of-the-same perspective. They also want to be healthy and financially secure. Changing demographics may contribute to new forms of inequality, such as the distribution of insecurity, emotional stress and ambivalence, which societies are currently ill equipped to remedy. Precarity in old age, exacerbated by lengthened statutory retirement ages, raises questions over availability and forms of work; plus, inadequate or unaffordable housing, care and support services also create sources of solidarity between younger and older adults. Solidarities arise from at least two sources – a common experience of uncertainty and a feeling that the contract between the government and its citizens has broken down, plus a lifetime-centred awareness that eroding rights in later life is eroding one's own future. Each of these issues suggests very different policy questions to those currently being considered both nationally and internationally.

Cultural adaptation for a long life

At root, cultural adaptation requires a different way of seeing the prospect of a long life and the possibilities for intergenerational connection. Different phases of the lifecourse are both distinctive and interconnected; they progress, perhaps through rhythm rather than in a linear, production-line manner. This places an emphasis on the complementary contributions that each phase brings to the intergenerational table, and we should not be afraid of recognising both continuities of identity and discontinuities of priority. We are the same people wanting to contribute different things at different times. To allow the special contribution of a long life to emerge requires resources and a certain faith that what arises may not be more of the same.

In order to get there, certain policy steps present themselves:

- First, we should audit the lifecourse. Each generational group brings something distinctive to the human project, arising from their lifecourse-based priorities. A clearly articulated view of the life tasks and priorities of each generation needs to move from tacit to explicit awareness. Unless proposed solutions answer lifetime-specific needs and priorities, people will not engage with them. Different perspectives might then be subject to popular democratic debate. What are your priorities? What do you want from a long life? What sort of intergenerational society do we want to build? How should resources be released to allow each generation to achieve this?
- Second, map the constituencies. We need to map where different age groups appear in society, especially with respect to decision-making processes. Age groups may be growing closer in size, but their distribution in social institutions

is currently unclear. Part of this process would concern a critical examination of how social institutions separate generations out from each other, making interconnection more difficult, and then the creation of forums for intergenerational reconnection.

• Third, take a lifetime view. Here a lifecourse perspective should come into effect, identifying the longitudinal consequences or scenarios that may result from particular forms of action or inaction. Ageing, in other words, is a long-burn issue, where people need predictability and reliability, requiring planning beyond electoral cycles. A lifetime view also emphasises the conditions that can prevent hazards to health and personal economic security arising.

• Fourth, let's road test the alternatives and create a series of cultural environments in which the potential of each phase of life can be given space to flourish and become recognised, both personally and socially. These spaces may occur naturally or be formally organised. We are only just beginning to inquire what the promise of a long life holds, for example, and we should increase the spaces in which to discover alternatives.

• Fifth, create a practical vision, through this discovery of prefigurative spaces that allow lifecourse-appropriate development and intergenerational complementarity to take place. This would involve a critical stepping back from narratives that have attempted to close down options and impose priorities from elsewhere. An identifying feature would be that experiment is facilitated through new forms of lifetime awareness, empathic understanding and positive intergenerational connection. As such, the vision would be able to contain experiences of in between-ness, where positive connections can be created and, with the passage of time, made manifest. They create, in other words, practical examples of generational intelligence.

Finally, and as a means to the ends identified above, we should rediscover interconnective government. Governmental policies and processes are often age specific, failing to address the effects of decisions on a wider generational milieu. Interconnection would apply equally to government agencies and departments where folios should practice dialogue between functions. This should include a special awareness of intergenerational consequences, generational proofing of policies and consultative structures specifically aimed at balancing age-specific and intergenerational priorities. The unfortunate history of government intervention on population ageing has been to try to fit emerging issues into preconceived and hastily concluded answers. These have characteristically relied on solutions imposed from other priority areas and based on a single age group perspective. In future, they might begin by identifying distinctive age priorities and follow through by connecting to intergenerational and lifetime perspectives.

The journey ahead

If the first phase of adaptation has been marked by a 'more of the same' response, filling the vacuum with priorities from elsewhere, and the second a facilitative and intergenerational response to the question of what to do with all those extra years, the third, which is only dimly visible on the horizon, may cause us to question some fundamental issues on the purpose of a long life, the contribution of older adults and a re-shaping of the lifecourse as a whole. The signposts are already there if we wish to follow them.

First would be to embrace the psycho-social discontinuities that occur as we age, rather than fear personal change. The mature half of adult life contains an awareness that we are not in fact immortal and have a limited time on this planet. This generates a set of new existential priorities that are only just becoming recognisable. It is not, then, simply that people wish they could spend more time in the workplace.

Second would be a rediscovery of the importance of generational intelligence. This would include both the ability to put oneself in the shoes of another generational group and to develop the skills for sustained negotiation between generational interests. The first steps noted above would enable us to evaluate the degree to which becoming conscious of self as part of a generation, the relative ability to put oneself in the position of other generations and the relative ability to negotiate between generational positions are taking place.

Taken together these two signposts would facilitate the discovery of each age group's contribution to social well-being and the development of complementary rather than competitive relations between those generations, in the workplace, in the family, in policy and in civil society. We have glimpses of these alternative rhythms in the differences between 'youthful' and 'mature' identities, age specific life tasks, changes in perspective, in 'gero-transcendence' and in 'generational intelligence'. They provide a starting point for the question of meaning in later life that is not solely contingent on economic materialism. The 'more of the same' offered by productivist solutions cannot answer these desires; rather it seeks to suppress them. We should, given this historical turn in age relations, see what it can tell us about the human condition, the ways we lead our lives and the kinds of futures we collectively desire.

If everybody really does want a long life, it is becoming clearer that few want to grow old as it is currently conceived. If the task is of cultural adaptation, then lasting solutions can be based on intergenerational complementarity. Policy should be less about work continuation versus re-invented retirement and more about allowing mature adults to develop multiple aspects of their identity and in so doing permit the emergence of lifecourse-specific contributions for the wider social good. The role of a progressive social policy would be to make available new social spaces in which these novel forms of age-based identities can develop. It would rest on a critique not only of physical space, but of temporal relations such as work-life balance across the lifecourse and the meanings attributed to different life phases. Sustainable solutions, ones that can stand the test of time and respect the life priorities of different generational groups, can then be negotiated as each party recognizes their own and the other's specific contribution. True cultural innovation would lie in the facilitation of new roles adapted to a long life, greater attention to generational interconnection, and discovering new ways of releasing age specific potential.

What's the answer to a long life? The answer is we don't fully know yet. New spaces and narratives will emerge that allow distinctive lifecourse and intergenerational priorities to come together, taking the best from the cultural raw material we have but forming something that is historically unprecedented. We are working towards a series of principles on which to judge whether emergent practices are in harmony with adult ageing and intergenerational sustainability or not. This is unknowing in a positive sense, in that the solutions will emerge from continuing generational exchange and from enhanced critical practice.

References

Biggs, S., & Lowenstein, A. (2011). Generational intelligence: A critical approach to age relations. New York, NY: Routledge.

Leime, A., Street, D., Vickerstaff, S., & Lorello, W. (2017). *Gender, ageing and extending working life: Cross-national perspectives*. Bristol: Policy Press.

Moulaert, T., & Garon, S. (Eds.). (2016). Age-friendly cities and communities in international comparison: Political lessons, scientific avenues, and democratic issues. New York, Springer.

Index

AAM *see* anti-ageing medicine (AAM)
abilities, increase in 36
abolishing ageing 112–113
Abramic belief systems 69, 72
abuse, social 138, 155
active ageing 3, 30–31
AD *see* Alzheimer's disease (AD)
Adam and Eve 69
affective relationships 151
affirmative prolongevism 121
A4M *see* American Academy of Anti-
Aging Medicine (A4M)
African Americans 65, 84
age/ageing: abolishing 112–113; active
3, 30–31; anti- 112–124; better
115; biological, interpreting 98–99;
chronological 105; deep old 97, 101;
delaying 112–113; facts of 4–5; fourth
100–101; functional 18, 57; global 1–2;
golden age of 75; intergenerational
14–26; natural 97–108, 101–104;
'not applying to us' 24; personal
14–26; positive 37; productive 30–31;
retirement and 33; slowing 118–119;
social 97–108; third 28, 32, 98,
100–101; unnatural, nature of 101–104;
wisdom and 89–91; work and health
related to 54; World Assemblies on
2; *see also* ageing/ageism and work;
ageing body; ageing related to belief
age-imperialism 9
ageing/ageism and work 29–30; abilities
and, increase in 36; from active to
productive 30–31; empowerment and
new 32–33; expectations and, increase
in 37–40
ageing body 97–108; biological ageing,
interpreting 98–99; natural, nature
of 101–104; naturalness, policy and

limitation on 104–107; sociology and
biology 99–101; unnatural, nature of
101–104
ageing related to belief 62–64; religions
and, major 71–75; strong associations
between 70–71; weak associations
between 70–71
ageism *see* ageing/ageism and work
agency, loss of 133
age-otherness 21–23
age-race wars 160
'aging enterprise' 133
Allah 73
Alzheimer's disease (AD) 128–129,
131–133, 139
ambivalence 35, 152–153
ambivalent relationships 151
American Academy of Anti-Aging
Medicine (A4M) 114–116
American Medical Association 114
AMP-NATCEM 37
Anderson, Perry 71
andropause 102
anger 91
Anthropocene 102
anti-ageing 112–124; abolishing aging
112–113; aspirational realties of 113–
114; bioscience and, relation between
116–118; cosmetics for 114; debates on
112; delaying aging 112–113; ideologies
of 123; longevity, commercialisation
of 119–120; medicine for 114; personal
consequences of 120–123; political
consequences of 120–123; prolongevism
and 113–114; science and 113–114;
social consequences of 120–123;
trajectory on, common 118–119; vision
of 114–116
anti-ageing medicine (AAM) 114–116, 133

Anti-Aging Medical News 115
ascending familialism 157
aspirational reality 113
aspirational realties of ageing 113–114
Atchley, Robert 17
attitudes between intergenerations
    158–161
Australian BSL Social Exclusion
    Monitor 7
Australian Institute for Family Studies 54,
    155
Australian Psychological Society 49, 51
awareness: lifetime-centred 169; present-
    centred 15, 24–25, 58, 124, 169, 171

Baby Boomers 34–36, 104
Bailey, S. 136–137
balance between life and work 54
Behuniak, S. 131, 135–136
being on time 84
belief: Abramic systems of 69, 72; aging
    related to 62–64; development stages of
    82; patterns of 80; religions and, major
    71–75; *see also* belief and spirituality
belief and spirituality: aging related
    to 62–64, 71–75; benefits of 64–66;
    lack and suffering related to 68–70;
    strong associations between 70–71;
    vulnerability and 66–68; weak
    associations between 70–71
better ageing 115
between-age thinking 15, 23–24, 26, 33,
    76, 142, 162, 169–171
Biggs, S. 16, 21, 22, 63, 82, 87, 137, 156,
    157, 160–161
biological ageing, interpreting 98–99
biological determinism 101
biological time 117
biology 99–101
bioscience and anti-ageing, relation
    between 116–118
BMW 36
British Medical Journal 155
Buddhism 62, 69, 72, 74–75
busy bodies 87
Butler, Bob 8

Calico 112
California Life Company 112
Canadian Prevalence Study 155
care and family 150
caregiver 155
care of the self 123

Carr, A. 137
Central Intelligence Agency (CIA) 4
centredness 24–26
Centre for Market Reform of Education 47
certainties, demographic 4–5
change/changing: continuity and 17–18,
    84–85; long life, prospect of 2–4;
    the narrative 30–31; non-spiritual
    explanations of 84
Christianity 62, 73
Christian thinking 70
chronological age 105
CIA *see* Central Intelligence Agency (CIA)
Club of Rome 5
cognitive functioning 51–52
'Coming of Age' (De Beauvoir) 18
commercialisation of longevity 119–120
commonsense reality 113
complex othering 21
conceptual journey to long life 8–10
Confucian teaching 74–75
conjunctive faith 82
conscious spirituality 81
consensual solidarity 151
continuity: change and 17–18, 84–85;
    discontinuity *vs.* 17–18; family and
    149–150; generational intelligence, from
    perspective of 17–18
Cornell Legacy Study 90
cosmetics for anti-ageing 114
critical approach to long life 8
cultural adaptation for long life 172–173
Cultural Revolution 154
cultural uncertainties surrounding long life
    6–8
culture and nature, boundary between 103

DAI *see* Dementia Alliance International
    (DAI)
debates on anti-ageing 112
De Beauvoir, Simone 18
deep old age 97, 101
dehumanisation 131
delaying ageing 112–113
dementia 128–142; as disease 131–134;
    first-person experiences of 140–141;
    narratives arising from 133–134;
    person-centred care for 134–135;
    pre-senile 132; from prolongevism to
    128–130; in the public domain 130–131;
    relationships and, emotional labour
    of 135–138; rights-based approach to
    141–142; risks associated with 138–139;

social images associated with 130; social inequality related to 138–139; structural factors related to 138–139; and zombie metaphor 131
Dementia Alliance International (DAI) 141
demographic certainties for long life 4–5
detached relationships 151
detachment 91
developmental psychology 85
discontinuity: continuity *vs.* 17–18; family and 149–150; gerotranscendence and power of 86; intergenerational relations and 88–89; positive 19, 23, 40, 58, 124, 161, 169–171; unthought knowns and positive 18–19
discordant relationships 151
disease, dementia as a 131–134
disengagement 87–88
downward familialism 157

early retirement 32
efficiency and personal care 137–138
ego psychology 82
Ehrlich, Paul 5
EIP-AHA *see* European Innovation Partnership on Active and Healthy Ageing (EIP-AHA)
Elder, G. H., Jr. 153–154
elder mistreatment 154–156
elders, feral 130
Eli 72
Elijah 72
Elisha 72
empowerment and new ageism 32–33
Erikson, E. H. 16, 18, 86–87, 89, 91, 97, 150
Estes, Caroll 8
European Commission 46
European Innovation Partnership on Active and Healthy Ageing (EIP-AHA) 48
European Parliament 139
European Working Group of People with Dementia (EWGPD) 141
European Year of Active Ageing and Intergenerational Solidarity 3
European Year of Active Ageing and Solidarity Between Generations 47
EWGPD *see* European Working Group of People with Dementia (EWGPD)
examination of life 83
exchanges between generations 156–158
expectations, increase in 37–40

facts of ageing 4–5
faithful narrative 35

familialism 157; *see also* family
family 148–162; care and 150; continuity and 149–150; discontinuity and 149–150; 'first half of life' achievements in 17; nuclear 156; relations between 148–149, 150–154; relationships within 151; social problems and 154–156; starting with 149–150; welfare as support for 158–159; *see also* generations/generational; intergenerations/intergenerational
feeling rules 136
fetishisation of work 40–41
final meanings 83
Financial Review 130
'first half of life' achievements in family 17
first-person experiences of dementia 140–141
Fontana, A. 136
'forgetful people' 137
fourth age 100–101
Freiden, Betty 31
Friedman, Rabbi 72
Friendly Society 32
functional ageing 18, 57
functional capacity model 115
functional solidarity 151
Furman, Dmitri 71

G8 Summit of 1997 30–31, 132
generational belonging 148–149
generational equity 160
generational intelligence 160, 169, 173; continuity from perspective of 17–18; gerotranscendence and 92, 174; importance of 174; lifecourse specificity and 15–16, 171; life priorities and 14; life's purpose and 16; low 160; negotiating 14–15; positive discontinuity and 19; relationships and 16; steps to 16
GenerationMe 34
generations/generational: exchanges between 156–158; intelligence 14–15; lifecourse specificity and 15–16; transfers between 156–158; work, differences in attitudes towards 33–36; *see also* family; intergenerations/intergenerational
Generations United USA 161
Generation X 34–36
Generation Y 34, 36
German Ageing Survey 40
gerotranscendence 85–88, 86, 92; generational intelligence and 92, 174

Gerotranscendence (Tornstam) 67
global ageing 1–2
global financial meltdown of 2008 120
Global Risks group 2
God 69–74, 83
'God to self' relationship 83
golden age of ageing 75
Golden Rule 75
Google 112
Grattan Institute 160
Great Depression 153

harmonious relationships 151
Harris, Gordon 72
health *see* work and health
Health and Retirement Study (HRS) 52
healthy life years (HLY) 48
hidden elements of identity 15–16
Hillel, Rabbi 75
Hinduism 62, 69, 72, 74
HLY *see* healthy life years (HLY)
Hochschild, A. 136
Hong Kong Christian Services 155
hope in life, search for 83
hormone replacement therapy (HRT)
    101–102
HRS *see* Health and Retirement Study
    (HRS)
humanism 63, 80
Hunter, P. V. 137–138

identity management 14–15; hidden
    elements of 15–16, 18; surface elements
    of 15–16, 18
ideologies of anti-ageing 123
ILO *see* International Labour Organisation
    (ILO)
independence and social inclusion 156–157
inequality 154, 160
inner life 70
insecure retirement 50
Institute of Economic Affairs 47
intelligence 90; *see also* generational
    intelligence
Intergenerational Foundation 160
intergenerations/intergenerational: ageing
    14–26; attitudes between 158–161;
    discontinuity and 88–89; politics
    between, rivalry of 158–161; rebalancing
    of 160; relations between 148–149;
    welfare between 158–161; *see also*
    family; generations/generational
International Labour Organisation (ILO)
    4, 7

intimate-but-distant relationships 151
Investing in Health report 106
Islam 62, 72–74

jaded by work 38
Jesus 75
Jewish Visions of Ageing (Friedman) 73
job satisfaction 34
Judaism 72–73
Jung, C. G. 10, 16–20, 85, 88–89, 97

Kairos 84
Kessler, L. 135–136
Kohli, Martin 9

lack 68–70, 88
Lancet 106
Lancet Neurology Commission 133
La Viellesse (De Beauvoir) 18
Legal Responsibility in Old Age 131
leisure time 52–53
Leviticus 75
LGBTI community 141
life: chances of 153; cultural adaptation for
    long 172–173; events in 84; examination
    of 83; extension of 115; hope in,
    search for 83; inner 70; priorities in 14;
    purpose of 16; relationships in, changes
    in 85; retirement for reclaiming 35;
    satisfaction in 86; self-enhancement and
    35; work and health, commodification
    related to 54–56; working 35, 46;
    working later in 28–29
lifecourse: generational belonging and
    148–149; generational intelligence and
    specificity of 15–16; Hinduism, stages
    of 81–82; naturalness and, connection
    between 97; specificity of 15–16,
    171; spiritual development and adult
    81–82; "Why" questions in 64; work
    and health, commodification related to
    56–57
lifespan, normal 105
lifetime-centred awareness 169
lifetime-centredness 24–26
lifetime thinking 24–25
liminality 63, 71
limitation on naturalness 104–107
linked lives 153
'live-longer, work-longer' solution 37
living in the past 25
"Living to 120 and beyond" survey 112
longevity: commercialisation of 119–120;
    dividend with 122; family, effects on

150; gap sin 122; narrative on 121; *see also* long life
long life 1–11; changing prospect of 2–4; conceptual journey to 8–10; critical approach to 8; cultural uncertainties surrounding 6–8; demographic certainties for 4–5; global ageing and 1–2; purpose of 10–11; *see also* longevity
loss of agency 133
loss of self 133
Lowenstein, A. 9, 16, 21, 160
low generational intelligence 160
Lutherans 69

'Madrid' statement 3
major religions 71–75
male menopause 102
malignant social psychology 135
Marmot Review 53
Marxism 63
McAdams, Dan 17
medicine for anti-ageing 114
memory 130–131
memory loss 130–131
menopause, male 102
Menzies, I. 136
midlife spirituality 84–85
Millennials 34–35
misery narrative 88
mistreatment of elders 154–156
moral queueing 123
'more of the same' response 11, 18

'nameless dread' 68–69
narrative 14–15; of ambivalence 35; changing the 30–31; dementia, arising from 133–134; of disaffection 35; faithful 35; hidden/surface elements of identity, impact on 19–21; on longevity 121; misery 88; present-centred 28–29; work and 28–31
natural ageing 97–108; nature of 101–104
natural athlete 102
natural lifespan 105
naturalness: lifecourse and notion of 97, 104; policy and limitation on 104–107
natural progression 88
natural selection 98
natural spirituality 81
natural teacher 102
nature and culture, boundary between 103
Nature Medicine 117, 120

negotiating generational intelligence 14–15
New Age Buddhism 87
new ageism 32–33
'New Age' lifestyles 116
'New Age' spiritual movements 80–81
New England Centenarian Study 117
New Testament 72
NHS 136
Noah 72
non-spiritual explanations of change 84
normal lifespan 105
normative solidarity 151
nuclear family 156

Oakland Growth Study 153
objective knowledge 99
obligatory relationships 151
OECD *see* Organisation for Economic Cooperation & Development (OECD)
'Old Age' (De Beauvoir) 18
Old Testament 72
Organisation for Economic Cooperation & Development (OECD) 4–5, 29, 31, 46, 48
organizational commitment 34
othering/otherness: age- 21–23; amplification of 131; complex 21; of other 129–130; positive 21–23, 41, 58, 148, 161, 171; process of 22; simple 21

personal ageing 14–26
personal care and efficiency 137–138
personal consequences of anti-ageing 120–123
person-centred care for dementia 134–135
personhood 134
person living with dementia (PLWD) 129–130, 129–132, 133–137, 139–142
Pew Research Center 159
Phillipson, Chris 8
pick and mix spirituality 81
PLWD *see* person living with dementia (PLWD)
policy: on naturalness 104–107; on work and health 46–48
political consequences of anti-ageing 120–123
politics between intergenerations, rivalry of 158–161
population bomb 5
positive ageing 37
positive discontinuity 18–19, 23, 40, 58, 124, 161, 169–171

positive disengagement 87
positive othering 21–23, 41, 58, 148, 161, 171
positive solitude 21, 86
possibility and time 80–81
pre-senile dementia 132
present-centred narrative 28–29
present-centredness 24–26
present-centred thinking/awareness 15, 24–25, 58, 124, 169, 171
productive ageing 30–31
prolongevism: affirmative 121; anti-ageing and 113–114; benefits of 112; to dementia 128–130; work and 129
psychological well-being 30
psychology 82, 85, 135
psychotherapy 83, 85
public domain, dementia in the 130–131
purpose of long life 10–11, 170

QALYs *see* quality adjusted life years (QALYs)
quality adjusted life years (QALYs) 105–106
quality of life following retirement 47
"Quality of Work, Wellbeing and Retirement" survey 50–51
Quran 73

reality 113
reasonable life span 105–106
Rejuvenation Research 114
relations/relationships: affective 151; ambivalent 151; categories of 83; and dementia, emotional labour of 135–138; detached 151; discordant 151; in family, changing approaches to 150–154; within family 151; between family and generations 148–149; generational intelligence and 16; 'God to self' 83; harmonious 151; between intergenerations 148–149; intimate-but-distant 151; in life, changes in 85; obligatory 151; social 151; tight-knit 151; of trust 155
religions, major 71–75
responsible self 123
restless experience of time 55–56
retirement 51–54; ageing and 33; Baby Boomers 37; early 32; insecure 50; quality of life following 47; for reclaiming life 35; transitioning to 52
rights-based approach to dementia 141–142

right time 84
risks associated with dementia 138–139
rituals for marking the passing of time 84

sacralisation of the self 80–81
Salzberg conference of 1982 31
Samuel 72
satisfaction in life 86
Science 117
science and anti-ageing 113–114
'science foreseeable' 118–119
SDG *see* Sustainable Development Goal (SDG)
self: care of the 123; loss of 133; responsible 123; sacralisation of the 80–81; sense of 85
'Self and suffering, a Buddhist-Christian conversation' (Ingram and Loy) 69
self and time 80–81
self-enhancement 35
self-esteem 34
selfhood, internal process of 100–101
'self to God' relationship 83
'self to life' relationship 83
'self to universe' relationship 83
self-transcendence 90
senility 131
sense of self 85
sensitising concept 85
sent-down generation 154
"shaking out" of the labour market 38
SHARE *see* Study of Health Ageing and Retirement in Europe (SHARE)
simple othering 21
slowing ageing 118–119
Smith, R. W. 136
social abuse 138, 155
social ageing 97–108
social consequences of anti-ageing 120–123
social gerontology 85
social images associated with dementia 130
social inclusion 87, 156–157
social inequality 138–139, 160
social isolation 86
social policy 152–153
social problems and family and generations 154–156
social psychology 135
social relationships 151
social well-being 30
sociology and biology 99–101

solidarity/solitude 151–152; consensual 151; functional 151; normative 151; positive 21, 86
Spira, Henry 67
spirituality 62–76; conscious 81; intelligence and, concepts of 90; lifecourse and 64, 81–82; as linear developmental process 84–85; midlife 84–85; natural 81; pick and mix 81; three-stage model of 82; wisdom and 90; *see also* belief and spirituality
'Stages of Faith' (Fowler) 82
Standing, Guy 7
'state of the heart' 74
state support 158–159
strong survivor effect 38
structural factors related to dementia 138–139
structural inequality 100
structural solidarity 151
Study of Health Ageing and Retirement in Europe (SHARE) 51
Successful Ageing 117
suffering 68–70
support bank 157
surface elements of identity 15–16
Sustainable Development Goal (SDG) 106
Swiftian nightmare 105

thinking/thoughts: between-age 15, 23–24, 26, 33, 76, 142, 162, 169–171; Christian 70; Confucian 74–75; lifetime 24–25; present-centred 15, 24–25, 58, 124, 169, 171; within-age 15, 23–24, 33, 124, 142, 170–171; within- and between-age 15, 23–24, 171
third age 28, 32, 98, 100–101
thoughts *see* thinking/thoughts
three-stage model of spirituality 82
tight-knit relationships 151
time/timing 84; being on 84; biological 117; leisure 52–53; possibility and 80–81; restless experience of 55–56; right 84; rituals for marking the passing of 84; self and 80–81; work and health, commodification related to 54–56, 56–57
trajectory on anti-ageing, common 118–119
transfers between generations 156–158
transitioning to retirement 52
'trentes glorieuses' 3, 104

trust, relationship of 155
Twenge, J. M. 34

unavoidable obligation 29
uncertainties, cultural 6–8
underemployed 50
UK Commission of Employment and Skills 49, 57
UK Department of Health 155
UK Trades Union Congress 47
United Nations Millennium Development Goals 161
United Nations Working Group on Older People 141–142
US Centers for Disease Control and Prevention 106, 128
US feminism 31
US Health and Retirement Study 52
US National Research Council 155
unnatural ageing, nature of 101–104
unthought knowns 18–19

Välitä Muista 137
Viagra 102
vision of anti-ageing 114–116
vulnerability 25, 66–68, 88, 98

welfare 158–161
well-being 30, 47, 90
'Whitehall' longitudinal study 38
WHO *see* World Health Organization (WHO)
"Why" questions in lifecourse 64
wisdom: ageing and 89–91; elderhood and 72; spirituality and 90
wise anger 91
within-age thinking 15, 23–24, 33, 124, 142, 170–171
work 28–41; ageing/ageism and 29–33, 36–40; balance between life and 54; cognitive functioning and 51–52; fetishisation of 40–41; 'first half of life' achievements in 17; generational differences in attitudes towards 33–36; imperialism of 54–55; jaded by 38; later in life 28–29; longevity and 122–123; narrative 28–31; solidarity and 152; well-being and, association between 47; *see also* work and health
work and health: ageing and 54; lifecourse time, commodification related to 56–57; life's time, commodification related

to 54–56; policy on 46–48; positives
vs. negatives on 46–58; relationship
between 48–51; retirement and 51–54
workers *vs.* professionals and creatives 38
Work Foundation 49
working life 35, 46
World Alzheimer's Report 128
World Assemblies on ageing 2
World Bank 4, 29, 106, 120
World Economic Forum 2

World Health Organization (WHO) 3–4,
30, 97, 115, 132–133, 155
WHO Action Plan on Non-Communicable
Diseases 106
WHO Global Dementia Observatory 132
World Report on Ageing and Health
(WHO) 106–107
World Social Protection Report 2014/15
(ILO) 4, 7
World War II 3, 104, 153